# Strain

Grower _____  Date _____

Acquired _____  $ _____

I0391110

---

Indica          Hybrid          Sativa

☐ Flower    ☐ Edible    ☐ Concentrate

Sweet
Fruity          Floral
Sour            Spicy
Earthy          Herbal
Woodsy

**Symptoms Relieved**

_____
_____
_____
_____

**Notes**

_____
_____
_____
_____
_____

| Effects | Strength | | | | |
|---|---|---|---|---|---|
| Peaceful | ○ | ○ | ○ | ○ | ○ |
| Sleepy | ○ | ○ | ○ | ○ | ○ |
| Pain Relief | ○ | ○ | ○ | ○ | ○ |
| Hungry | ○ | ○ | ○ | ○ | ○ |
| Uplifted | ○ | ○ | ○ | ○ | ○ |
| Creative | ○ | ○ | ○ | ○ | ○ |

Ratings ☆ ☆ ☆ ☆ ☆

# Strain

Grower _____    Date _____

Acquired _____    $ _____

| Indica | Hybrid | Sativa |

☐ Flower    ☐ Edible    ☐ Concentrate

**Symptoms Relieved**

_____
_____
_____
_____

Sweet / Fruity / Floral / Sour / Spicy / Earthy / Woodsy / Herbal

**Notes**

_____
_____
_____
_____
_____
_____

| Effects | Strength |
|---|---|
| Peaceful | ○ ○ ○ ○ ○ |
| Sleepy | ○ ○ ○ ○ ○ |
| Pain Relief | ○ ○ ○ ○ ○ |
| Hungry | ○ ○ ○ ○ ○ |
| Uplifted | ○ ○ ○ ○ ○ |
| Creative | ○ ○ ○ ○ ○ |

**Ratings** ☆ ☆ ☆ ☆ ☆

# Strain

Grower _____  Date _____

Acquired _____  $ _____

| Indica | Hybrid | Sativa |

☐ Flower  ☐ Edible  ☐ Concentrate

**Symptoms Relieved**

_____
_____
_____
_____

Flavor wheel: Sweet, Floral, Spicy, Herbal, Woodsy, Earthy, Sour, Fruity

**Notes**

_____
_____
_____
_____
_____

| Effects | Strength | | | | |
|---|---|---|---|---|---|
| Peaceful | ○ | ○ | ○ | ○ | ○ |
| Sleepy | ○ | ○ | ○ | ○ | ○ |
| Pain Relief | ○ | ○ | ○ | ○ | ○ |
| Hungry | ○ | ○ | ○ | ○ | ○ |
| Uplifted | ○ | ○ | ○ | ○ | ○ |
| Creative | ○ | ○ | ○ | ○ | ○ |

**Ratings** ☆ ☆ ☆ ☆ ☆

# Strain

Grower _____ Date _____

Acquired _____ $ _____

| Indica | Hybrid | Sativa |

☐ Flower   ☐ Edible   ☐ Concentrate

**Symptoms Relieved**

_____
_____
_____
_____
_____

Sweet · Fruity · Floral · Sour · Spicy · Earthy · Woodsy · Herbal

**Notes**

_____
_____
_____
_____
_____
_____
_____

| Effects | Strength | | | | |
|---|---|---|---|---|---|
| Peaceful | ○ | ○ | ○ | ○ | ○ |
| Sleepy | ○ | ○ | ○ | ○ | ○ |
| Pain Relief | ○ | ○ | ○ | ○ | ○ |
| Hungry | ○ | ○ | ○ | ○ | ○ |
| Uplifted | ○ | ○ | ○ | ○ | ○ |
| Creative | ○ | ○ | ○ | ○ | ○ |

**Ratings** ☆ ☆ ☆ ☆ ☆

# Strain

Grower _____  Date _____

Acquired _____  $ _____

| Indica | Hybrid | Sativa |

☐ Flower  ☐ Edible  ☐ Concentrate

Sweet · Floral · Spicy · Herbal · Woodsy · Earthy · Sour · Fruity

**Symptoms Relieved**

_____
_____
_____
_____
_____

**Notes**

_____
_____
_____
_____
_____
_____

| Effects | Strength | | | | |
|---|---|---|---|---|---|
| Peaceful | ○ | ○ | ○ | ○ | ○ |
| Sleepy | ○ | ○ | ○ | ○ | ○ |
| Pain Relief | ○ | ○ | ○ | ○ | ○ |
| Hungry | ○ | ○ | ○ | ○ | ○ |
| Uplifted | ○ | ○ | ○ | ○ | ○ |
| Creative | ○ | ○ | ○ | ○ | ○ |

**Ratings** ☆ ☆ ☆ ☆ ☆

# Strain

Grower _____    Date _____

Acquired _____    $ _____

| Indica | Hybrid | Sativa |

☐ Flower   ☐ Edible   ☐ Concentrate

**Symptoms Relieved**

_____
_____
_____
_____
_____

Sweet · Floral · Spicy · Herbal · Woodsy · Earthy · Sour · Fruity

**Notes**

_____
_____
_____
_____
_____
_____

| Effects | Strength | | | | |
|---|---|---|---|---|---|
| Peaceful | ○ | ○ | ○ | ○ | ○ |
| Sleepy | ○ | ○ | ○ | ○ | ○ |
| Pain Relief | ○ | ○ | ○ | ○ | ○ |
| Hungry | ○ | ○ | ○ | ○ | ○ |
| Uplifted | ○ | ○ | ○ | ○ | ○ |
| Creative | ○ | ○ | ○ | ○ | ○ |

**Ratings** ☆ ☆ ☆ ☆ ☆

# Strain

Grower _____  Date _____

Acquired _____  $ _____

| Indica | Hybrid | Sativa |

☐ Flower   ☐ Edible   ☐ Concentrate

**Symptoms Relieved**

_____
_____
_____
_____

Sweet · Floral · Spicy · Herbal · Woodsy · Earthy · Sour · Fruity

**Notes**

_____
_____
_____
_____
_____
_____

| Effects | Strength | | | | |
|---|---|---|---|---|---|
| Peaceful | ○ | ○ | ○ | ○ | ○ |
| Sleepy | ○ | ○ | ○ | ○ | ○ |
| Pain Relief | ○ | ○ | ○ | ○ | ○ |
| Hungry | ○ | ○ | ○ | ○ | ○ |
| Uplifted | ○ | ○ | ○ | ○ | ○ |
| Creative | ○ | ○ | ○ | ○ | ○ |

**Ratings** ☆ ☆ ☆ ☆ ☆

# Strain

Grower _____    Date _____

Acquired _____    $ _____

| Indica | Hybrid | Sativa |

☐ Flower   ☐ Edible   ☐ Concentrate

**Symptoms Relieved**

_____
_____
_____
_____
_____

Sweet · Fruity · Floral · Sour · Spicy · Earthy · Woodsy · Herbal

**Notes**

_____
_____
_____
_____
_____
_____

| Effects | Strength | | | | |
|---|---|---|---|---|---|
| Peaceful | ○ | ○ | ○ | ○ | ○ |
| Sleepy | ○ | ○ | ○ | ○ | ○ |
| Pain Relief | ○ | ○ | ○ | ○ | ○ |
| Hungry | ○ | ○ | ○ | ○ | ○ |
| Uplifted | ○ | ○ | ○ | ○ | ○ |
| Creative | ○ | ○ | ○ | ○ | ○ |

**Ratings** ☆ ☆ ☆ ☆ ☆

# Strain

Grower _____     Date _____

Acquired _____     $ _____

| Indica | Hybrid | Sativa |

☐ Flower  ☐ Edible  ☐ Concentrate

**Symptoms Relieved**

_____
_____
_____
_____
_____

Sweet · Floral · Spicy · Herbal · Woodsy · Earthy · Sour · Fruity

**Notes**

_____
_____
_____
_____
_____
_____
_____

| Effects | Strength | | | | |
|---|---|---|---|---|---|
| Peaceful | ○ | ○ | ○ | ○ | ○ |
| Sleepy | ○ | ○ | ○ | ○ | ○ |
| Pain Relief | ○ | ○ | ○ | ○ | ○ |
| Hungry | ○ | ○ | ○ | ○ | ○ |
| Uplifted | ○ | ○ | ○ | ○ | ○ |
| Creative | ○ | ○ | ○ | ○ | ○ |

**Ratings** ☆ ☆ ☆ ☆ ☆

# Strain

Grower _____   Date _____

Acquired _____   $ _____

| Indica | Hybrid | Sativa |

☐ Flower  ☐ Edible  ☐ Concentrate

**Symptoms Relieved**

_____
_____
_____
_____
_____

Sweet · Floral · Spicy · Herbal · Woodsy · Earthy · Sour · Fruity

**Notes**

_____
_____
_____
_____
_____
_____

| Effects | Strength | | | | |
|---|---|---|---|---|---|
| Peaceful | ○ | ○ | ○ | ○ | ○ |
| Sleepy | ○ | ○ | ○ | ○ | ○ |
| Pain Relief | ○ | ○ | ○ | ○ | ○ |
| Hungry | ○ | ○ | ○ | ○ | ○ |
| Uplifted | ○ | ○ | ○ | ○ | ○ |
| Creative | ○ | ○ | ○ | ○ | ○ |

**Ratings** ☆ ☆ ☆ ☆ ☆

# Strain

Grower _____    Date _____

Acquired _____    $ _____

| Indica | Hybrid | Sativa |

☐ Flower  ☐ Edible  ☐ Concentrate

**Symptoms Relieved**

_____
_____
_____
_____
_____

Flavor wheel: Sweet, Floral, Spicy, Herbal, Woodsy, Earthy, Sour, Fruity

**Notes**

_____
_____
_____
_____
_____
_____
_____

| Effects | Strength | | | | |
|---|---|---|---|---|---|
| Peaceful | ○ | ○ | ○ | ○ | ○ |
| Sleepy | ○ | ○ | ○ | ○ | ○ |
| Pain Relief | ○ | ○ | ○ | ○ | ○ |
| Hungry | ○ | ○ | ○ | ○ | ○ |
| Uplifted | ○ | ○ | ○ | ○ | ○ |
| Creative | ○ | ○ | ○ | ○ | ○ |

**Ratings** ☆ ☆ ☆ ☆ ☆

# Strain

Grower _____  Date _____

Acquired _____  $ _____

| Indica | Hybrid | Sativa |

☐ Flower  ☐ Edible  ☐ Concentrate

## Symptoms Relieved

_____
_____
_____
_____

Sweet · Fruity · Floral · Sour · Spicy · Earthy · Herbal · Woodsy

## Notes

_____
_____
_____
_____
_____

| Effects | Strength |
|---|---|
| Peaceful | ○ ○ ○ ○ ○ |
| Sleepy | ○ ○ ○ ○ ○ |
| Pain Relief | ○ ○ ○ ○ ○ |
| Hungry | ○ ○ ○ ○ ○ |
| Uplifted | ○ ○ ○ ○ ○ |
| Creative | ○ ○ ○ ○ ○ |

**Ratings** ☆ ☆ ☆ ☆ ☆

# Strain

Grower _____  Date _____

Acquired _____  $ _____

| Indica | Hybrid | Sativa |

☐ Flower  ☐ Edible  ☐ Concentrate

Sweet · Floral · Spicy · Herbal · Woodsy · Earthy · Sour · Fruity

## Symptoms Relieved

_____
_____
_____
_____
_____

## Notes

_____
_____
_____
_____
_____
_____

| Effects | Strength |
|---|---|
| Peaceful | ○ ○ ○ ○ ○ |
| Sleepy | ○ ○ ○ ○ ○ |
| Pain Relief | ○ ○ ○ ○ ○ |
| Hungry | ○ ○ ○ ○ ○ |
| Uplifted | ○ ○ ○ ○ ○ |
| Creative | ○ ○ ○ ○ ○ |

**Ratings** ☆ ☆ ☆ ☆ ☆

# Strain

Grower _____  Date _____

Acquired _____  $ _____

| Indica | Hybrid | Sativa |

☐ Flower   ☐ Edible   ☐ Concentrate

**Symptoms Relieved**

_____
_____
_____
_____
_____

Flavor wheel: Sweet, Floral, Spicy, Herbal, Woodsy, Earthy, Sour, Fruity

**Notes**

_____
_____
_____
_____
_____
_____

| Effects | Strength |
|---|---|
| Peaceful | ○ ○ ○ ○ ○ |
| Sleepy | ○ ○ ○ ○ ○ |
| Pain Relief | ○ ○ ○ ○ ○ |
| Hungry | ○ ○ ○ ○ ○ |
| Uplifted | ○ ○ ○ ○ ○ |
| Creative | ○ ○ ○ ○ ○ |

**Ratings** ☆ ☆ ☆ ☆ ☆

# Strain

Grower _____    Date _____

Acquired _____    $ _____

| Indica | Hybrid | Sativa |

☐ Flower  ☐ Edible  ☐ Concentrate

**Symptoms Relieved**

_____

_____

_____

_____

Flavor wheel: Sweet, Floral, Spicy, Herbal, Woodsy, Earthy, Sour, Fruity

**Notes**

_____

_____

_____

_____

_____

| Effects | Strength | | | | |
|---|---|---|---|---|---|
| Peaceful | ○ | ○ | ○ | ○ | ○ |
| Sleepy | ○ | ○ | ○ | ○ | ○ |
| Pain Relief | ○ | ○ | ○ | ○ | ○ |
| Hungry | ○ | ○ | ○ | ○ | ○ |
| Uplifted | ○ | ○ | ○ | ○ | ○ |
| Creative | ○ | ○ | ○ | ○ | ○ |

**Ratings** ☆ ☆ ☆ ☆ ☆

# Strain

Grower _____  Date _____

Acquired _____  $ _____

| Indica | Hybrid | Sativa |

☐ Flower   ☐ Edible   ☐ Concentrate

**Symptoms Relieved**

_____
_____
_____
_____
_____

Sweet · Fruity · Floral · Sour · Spicy · Earthy · Woodsy · Herbal

**Notes**

_____
_____
_____
_____
_____
_____

| Effects | Strength | | | | |
|---|---|---|---|---|---|
| Peaceful | ○ | ○ | ○ | ○ | ○ |
| Sleepy | ○ | ○ | ○ | ○ | ○ |
| Pain Relief | ○ | ○ | ○ | ○ | ○ |
| Hungry | ○ | ○ | ○ | ○ | ○ |
| Uplifted | ○ | ○ | ○ | ○ | ○ |
| Creative | ○ | ○ | ○ | ○ | ○ |

**Ratings** ☆ ☆ ☆ ☆ ☆

# Strain

Grower _____    Date _____

Acquired _____    $ _____

| Indica | Hybrid | Sativa |

☐ Flower   ☐ Edible   ☐ Concentrate

**Symptoms Relieved**

_____
_____
_____
_____
_____

Sweet · Floral · Spicy · Herbal · Woodsy · Earthy · Sour · Fruity

**Notes**

_____
_____
_____
_____
_____
_____

| Effects | Strength |
|---|---|
| Peaceful | ○ ○ ○ ○ ○ |
| Sleepy | ○ ○ ○ ○ ○ |
| Pain Relief | ○ ○ ○ ○ ○ |
| Hungry | ○ ○ ○ ○ ○ |
| Uplifted | ○ ○ ○ ○ ○ |
| Creative | ○ ○ ○ ○ ○ |

**Ratings** ☆ ☆ ☆ ☆ ☆

# Strain

Grower _____   Date _____

Acquired _____   $ _____

| Indica | Hybrid | Sativa |

☐ Flower    ☐ Edible    ☐ Concentrate

**Symptoms Relieved**

_____
_____
_____
_____

Sweet · Fruity · Floral · Sour · Spicy · Earthy · Woodsy · Herbal

**Notes**

_____
_____
_____
_____
_____

| Effects | Strength | | | | |
|---|---|---|---|---|---|
| Peaceful | ○ | ○ | ○ | ○ | ○ |
| Sleepy | ○ | ○ | ○ | ○ | ○ |
| Pain Relief | ○ | ○ | ○ | ○ | ○ |
| Hungry | ○ | ○ | ○ | ○ | ○ |
| Uplifted | ○ | ○ | ○ | ○ | ○ |
| Creative | ○ | ○ | ○ | ○ | ○ |

**Ratings** ☆ ☆ ☆ ☆ ☆

# Strain

Grower _____   Date _____

Acquired _____   $ _____

| Indica | Hybrid | Sativa |

☐ Flower   ☐ Edible   ☐ Concentrate

Sweet · Floral · Spicy · Herbal · Woodsy · Earthy · Sour · Fruity

**Symptoms Relieved**

_____
_____
_____
_____
_____

**Notes**

_____
_____
_____
_____
_____
_____

| Effects | Strength | | | | |
|---|---|---|---|---|---|
| Peaceful | ○ | ○ | ○ | ○ | ○ |
| Sleepy | ○ | ○ | ○ | ○ | ○ |
| Pain Relief | ○ | ○ | ○ | ○ | ○ |
| Hungry | ○ | ○ | ○ | ○ | ○ |
| Uplifted | ○ | ○ | ○ | ○ | ○ |
| Creative | ○ | ○ | ○ | ○ | ○ |

**Ratings** ☆ ☆ ☆ ☆ ☆

# Strain

Grower _____  Date _____

Acquired _____  $ _____

|   Indica   |   Hybrid   |   Sativa   |

☐ Flower   ☐ Edible   ☐ Concentrate

**Symptoms Relieved**

_____
_____
_____
_____
_____

Sweet · Fruity · Floral · Sour · Spicy · Earthy · Woodsy · Herbal

**Notes**

_____
_____
_____
_____
_____
_____

| Effects | Strength | | | | |
|---|---|---|---|---|---|
| Peaceful | ○ | ○ | ○ | ○ | ○ |
| Sleepy | ○ | ○ | ○ | ○ | ○ |
| Pain Relief | ○ | ○ | ○ | ○ | ○ |
| Hungry | ○ | ○ | ○ | ○ | ○ |
| Uplifted | ○ | ○ | ○ | ○ | ○ |
| Creative | ○ | ○ | ○ | ○ | ○ |

**Ratings** ☆ ☆ ☆ ☆ ☆

# Strain

Grower _____  Date _____

Acquired _____  $ _____

| Indica | Hybrid | Sativa |

☐ Flower   ☐ Edible   ☐ Concentrate

**Symptoms Relieved**

_____
_____
_____
_____
_____

Sweet · Floral · Spicy · Herbal · Woodsy · Earthy · Sour · Fruity

**Notes**

_____
_____
_____
_____
_____
_____

| Effects | Strength | | | | |
|---|---|---|---|---|---|
| Peaceful | ○ | ○ | ○ | ○ | ○ |
| Sleepy | ○ | ○ | ○ | ○ | ○ |
| Pain Relief | ○ | ○ | ○ | ○ | ○ |
| Hungry | ○ | ○ | ○ | ○ | ○ |
| Uplifted | ○ | ○ | ○ | ○ | ○ |
| Creative | ○ | ○ | ○ | ○ | ○ |

**Ratings** ☆ ☆ ☆ ☆ ☆

# Strain

Grower _____  Date _____

Acquired _____  $ _____

| Indica | Hybrid | Sativa |

☐ Flower  ☐ Edible  ☐ Concentrate

**Symptoms Relieved**

_____
_____
_____
_____
_____

Sweet • Floral • Spicy • Herbal • Woodsy • Earthy • Sour • Fruity

**Notes**

_____
_____
_____
_____
_____
_____

| Effects | Strength | | | | |
|---|---|---|---|---|---|
| Peaceful | ○ | ○ | ○ | ○ | ○ |
| Sleepy | ○ | ○ | ○ | ○ | ○ |
| Pain Relief | ○ | ○ | ○ | ○ | ○ |
| Hungry | ○ | ○ | ○ | ○ | ○ |
| Uplifted | ○ | ○ | ○ | ○ | ○ |
| Creative | ○ | ○ | ○ | ○ | ○ |

**Ratings** ☆ ☆ ☆ ☆ ☆

# Strain

Grower _____  Date _____

Acquired _____  $ _____

| Indica | Hybrid | Sativa |

☐ Flower  ☐ Edible  ☐ Concentrate

**Symptoms Relieved**
_____
_____
_____
_____
_____

Sweet · Floral · Spicy · Herbal · Woodsy · Earthy · Sour · Fruity

**Notes**
_____
_____
_____
_____
_____
_____

| Effects | Strength | | | | |
|---|---|---|---|---|---|
| Peaceful | ○ | ○ | ○ | ○ | ○ |
| Sleepy | ○ | ○ | ○ | ○ | ○ |
| Pain Relief | ○ | ○ | ○ | ○ | ○ |
| Hungry | ○ | ○ | ○ | ○ | ○ |
| Uplifted | ○ | ○ | ○ | ○ | ○ |
| Creative | ○ | ○ | ○ | ○ | ○ |

**Ratings** ☆ ☆ ☆ ☆ ☆

# Strain

Grower _____  Date _____

Acquired _____  $ _____

|  Indica | Hybrid | Sativa |

☐ Flower   ☐ Edible   ☐ Concentrate

Sweet
Fruity        Floral
Sour          Spicy
Earthy        Herbal
Woodsy

## Symptoms Relieved
_____
_____
_____
_____

## Notes
_____
_____
_____
_____
_____
_____

| Effects | Strength |
|---|---|
| Peaceful | ○ ○ ○ ○ ○ |
| Sleepy | ○ ○ ○ ○ ○ |
| Pain Relief | ○ ○ ○ ○ ○ |
| Hungry | ○ ○ ○ ○ ○ |
| Uplifted | ○ ○ ○ ○ ○ |
| Creative | ○ ○ ○ ○ ○ |

**Ratings** ☆ ☆ ☆ ☆ ☆

# Strain

Grower _____  Date _____

Acquired _____  $ _____

| Indica | Hybrid | Sativa |

☐ Flower  ☐ Edible  ☐ Concentrate

Sweet
Fruity    Floral
Sour    Spicy
Earthy    Herbal
Woodsy

**Symptoms Relieved**

_____
_____
_____
_____
_____

**Notes**

_____
_____
_____
_____
_____
_____

| Effects | Strength | | | | |
|---|---|---|---|---|---|
| Peaceful | ○ | ○ | ○ | ○ | ○ |
| Sleepy | ○ | ○ | ○ | ○ | ○ |
| Pain Relief | ○ | ○ | ○ | ○ | ○ |
| Hungry | ○ | ○ | ○ | ○ | ○ |
| Uplifted | ○ | ○ | ○ | ○ | ○ |
| Creative | ○ | ○ | ○ | ○ | ○ |

**Ratings** ☆ ☆ ☆ ☆ ☆

# Strain

Grower _____ Date _____

Acquired _____ $ _____

| Indica | Hybrid | Sativa |

☐ Flower  ☐ Edible  ☐ Concentrate

**Symptoms Relieved**

_____
_____
_____
_____

Sweet / Floral / Spicy / Herbal / Woodsy / Earthy / Sour / Fruity

**Notes**

_____
_____
_____
_____
_____

| Effects | Strength |
|---|---|
| Peaceful | ○ ○ ○ ○ ○ |
| Sleepy | ○ ○ ○ ○ ○ |
| Pain Relief | ○ ○ ○ ○ ○ |
| Hungry | ○ ○ ○ ○ ○ |
| Uplifted | ○ ○ ○ ○ ○ |
| Creative | ○ ○ ○ ○ ○ |

**Ratings** ☆ ☆ ☆ ☆ ☆

# Strain

Grower _____  Date _____

Acquired _____  $ _____

| Indica | Hybrid | Sativa |

☐ Flower   ☐ Edible   ☐ Concentrate

**Symptoms Relieved**

_____
_____
_____
_____
_____

Sweet · Fruity · Floral · Sour · Spicy · Earthy · Herbal · Woodsy

**Notes**

_____
_____
_____
_____
_____
_____

| Effects | Strength | | | | |
|---|---|---|---|---|---|
| Peaceful | ○ | ○ | ○ | ○ | ○ |
| Sleepy | ○ | ○ | ○ | ○ | ○ |
| Pain Relief | ○ | ○ | ○ | ○ | ○ |
| Hungry | ○ | ○ | ○ | ○ | ○ |
| Uplifted | ○ | ○ | ○ | ○ | ○ |
| Creative | ○ | ○ | ○ | ○ | ○ |

**Ratings** ☆ ☆ ☆ ☆ ☆

# Strain

Grower _____  Date _____

Acquired _____  $ _____

| Indica | Hybrid | Sativa |

☐ Flower  ☐ Edible  ☐ Concentrate

**Symptoms Relieved**

_____
_____
_____
_____

Sweet · Fruity · Floral · Sour · Spicy · Earthy · Woodsy · Herbal

**Notes**

_____
_____
_____
_____
_____

| Effects | Strength |
|---|---|
| Peaceful | ○ ○ ○ ○ ○ |
| Sleepy | ○ ○ ○ ○ ○ |
| Pain Relief | ○ ○ ○ ○ ○ |
| Hungry | ○ ○ ○ ○ ○ |
| Uplifted | ○ ○ ○ ○ ○ |
| Creative | ○ ○ ○ ○ ○ |

**Ratings** ☆ ☆ ☆ ☆ ☆

# Strain

Grower _____   Date _____

Acquired _____   $ _____

| Indica | Hybrid | Sativa |

☐ Flower  ☐ Edible  ☐ Concentrate

Sweet
Fruity    Floral
Sour      Spicy
Earthy    Herbal
Woodsy

**Symptoms Relieved**

_____
_____
_____
_____
_____

**Notes**

_____
_____
_____
_____
_____
_____

| **Effects** | **Strength** | | | | |
|---|---|---|---|---|---|
| Peaceful | ○ | ○ | ○ | ○ | ○ |
| Sleepy | ○ | ○ | ○ | ○ | ○ |
| Pain Relief | ○ | ○ | ○ | ○ | ○ |
| Hungry | ○ | ○ | ○ | ○ | ○ |
| Uplifted | ○ | ○ | ○ | ○ | ○ |
| Creative | ○ | ○ | ○ | ○ | ○ |

**Ratings** ☆ ☆ ☆ ☆ ☆

# Strain

Grower _____  Date _____

Acquired _____  $ _____

Indica        Hybrid        Sativa

☐ Flower   ☐ Edible   ☐ Concentrate

**Symptoms Relieved**
_____
_____
_____
_____
_____

Sweet · Floral · Spicy · Herbal · Woodsy · Earthy · Sour · Fruity

**Notes**
_____
_____
_____
_____
_____
_____
_____

| Effects | Strength | | | | |
|---|---|---|---|---|---|
| Peaceful | ○ | ○ | ○ | ○ | ○ |
| Sleepy | ○ | ○ | ○ | ○ | ○ |
| Pain Relief | ○ | ○ | ○ | ○ | ○ |
| Hungry | ○ | ○ | ○ | ○ | ○ |
| Uplifted | ○ | ○ | ○ | ○ | ○ |
| Creative | ○ | ○ | ○ | ○ | ○ |

**Ratings** ☆ ☆ ☆ ☆ ☆

# Strain

Grower _____  Date _____

Acquired _____  $ _____

| Indica | Hybrid | Sativa |

☐ Flower  ☐ Edible  ☐ Concentrate

**Symptoms Relieved**

_____
_____
_____
_____

Sweet · Fruity · Floral · Sour · Spicy · Earthy · Herbal · Woodsy

**Notes**

_____
_____
_____
_____
_____

| Effects | Strength | | | | |
|---|---|---|---|---|---|
| Peaceful | ○ | ○ | ○ | ○ | ○ |
| Sleepy | ○ | ○ | ○ | ○ | ○ |
| Pain Relief | ○ | ○ | ○ | ○ | ○ |
| Hungry | ○ | ○ | ○ | ○ | ○ |
| Uplifted | ○ | ○ | ○ | ○ | ○ |
| Creative | ○ | ○ | ○ | ○ | ○ |

Ratings ☆ ☆ ☆ ☆ ☆

# Strain

Grower _____  Date _____

Acquired _____  $ _____

| Indica | Hybrid | Sativa |

☐ Flower  ☐ Edible  ☐ Concentrate

**Symptoms Relieved**

_____
_____
_____
_____
_____

Sweet / Fruity / Floral / Sour / Spicy / Earthy / Woodsy / Herbal

**Notes**

_____
_____
_____
_____
_____
_____

| Effects | Strength | | | | |
|---|---|---|---|---|---|
| Peaceful | ○ | ○ | ○ | ○ | ○ |
| Sleepy | ○ | ○ | ○ | ○ | ○ |
| Pain Relief | ○ | ○ | ○ | ○ | ○ |
| Hungry | ○ | ○ | ○ | ○ | ○ |
| Uplifted | ○ | ○ | ○ | ○ | ○ |
| Creative | ○ | ○ | ○ | ○ | ○ |

**Ratings** ☆ ☆ ☆ ☆ ☆

# Strain

Grower _____  Date _____

Acquired _____  $ _____

| Indica | Hybrid | Sativa |

☐ Flower  ☐ Edible  ☐ Concentrate

Sweet
Fruity      Floral
Sour         Spicy
Earthy      Herbal
Woodsy

**Symptoms Relieved**

_____
_____
_____
_____
_____

**Notes**

_____
_____
_____
_____
_____
_____

| Effects | Strength |
|---|---|
| Peaceful | ○ ○ ○ ○ ○ |
| Sleepy | ○ ○ ○ ○ ○ |
| Pain Relief | ○ ○ ○ ○ ○ |
| Hungry | ○ ○ ○ ○ ○ |
| Uplifted | ○ ○ ○ ○ ○ |
| Creative | ○ ○ ○ ○ ○ |

**Ratings** ☆ ☆ ☆ ☆ ☆

# Strain

Grower _____  Date _____

Acquired _____  $ _____

| Indica | Hybrid | Sativa |

☐ Flower  ☐ Edible  ☐ Concentrate

**Symptoms Relieved**

_____
_____
_____
_____

Sweet / Fruity / Floral / Sour / Spicy / Earthy / Woodsy / Herbal

**Notes**

_____
_____
_____
_____
_____
_____

| Effects | Strength |
|---|---|
| Peaceful | ○ ○ ○ ○ ○ |
| Sleepy | ○ ○ ○ ○ ○ |
| Pain Relief | ○ ○ ○ ○ ○ |
| Hungry | ○ ○ ○ ○ ○ |
| Uplifted | ○ ○ ○ ○ ○ |
| Creative | ○ ○ ○ ○ ○ |

**Ratings** ☆ ☆ ☆ ☆ ☆

# Strain

Grower _____    Date _____

Acquired _____    $ _____

| Indica | Hybrid | Sativa |

☐ Flower   ☐ Edible   ☐ Concentrate

**Symptoms Relieved**

_____
_____
_____
_____
_____

Flavor wheel: Sweet, Floral, Spicy, Herbal, Woodsy, Earthy, Sour, Fruity

**Notes**

_____
_____
_____
_____
_____
_____

| Effects | Strength | | | | |
|---|---|---|---|---|---|
| Peaceful | ○ | ○ | ○ | ○ | ○ |
| Sleepy | ○ | ○ | ○ | ○ | ○ |
| Pain Relief | ○ | ○ | ○ | ○ | ○ |
| Hungry | ○ | ○ | ○ | ○ | ○ |
| Uplifted | ○ | ○ | ○ | ○ | ○ |
| Creative | ○ | ○ | ○ | ○ | ○ |

**Ratings** ☆ ☆ ☆ ☆ ☆

# Strain

Grower _____  Date _____
Acquired _____  $ _____

|  Indica  |  Hybrid  |  Sativa  |

☐ Flower   ☐ Edible   ☐ Concentrate

**Symptoms Relieved**
_____
_____
_____
_____

Sweet · Floral · Spicy · Herbal · Woodsy · Earthy · Sour · Fruity

**Notes**
_____
_____
_____
_____
_____
_____

| Effects | Strength | | | | |
|---|---|---|---|---|---|
| Peaceful | ○ | ○ | ○ | ○ | ○ |
| Sleepy | ○ | ○ | ○ | ○ | ○ |
| Pain Relief | ○ | ○ | ○ | ○ | ○ |
| Hungry | ○ | ○ | ○ | ○ | ○ |
| Uplifted | ○ | ○ | ○ | ○ | ○ |
| Creative | ○ | ○ | ○ | ○ | ○ |

**Ratings** ☆ ☆ ☆ ☆ ☆

# Strain

Grower _____  Date _____

Acquired _____  $ _____

|  Indica           Hybrid            Sativa  |

☐ Flower   ☐ Edible   ☐ Concentrate

**Symptoms Relieved**

_____
_____
_____
_____
_____

Flavor wheel: Sweet, Floral, Spicy, Herbal, Woodsy, Earthy, Sour, Fruity

**Notes**

_____
_____
_____
_____
_____
_____

| Effects | Strength | | | | |
|---|---|---|---|---|---|
| Peaceful | ○ | ○ | ○ | ○ | ○ |
| Sleepy | ○ | ○ | ○ | ○ | ○ |
| Pain Relief | ○ | ○ | ○ | ○ | ○ |
| Hungry | ○ | ○ | ○ | ○ | ○ |
| Uplifted | ○ | ○ | ○ | ○ | ○ |
| Creative | ○ | ○ | ○ | ○ | ○ |

**Ratings** ☆ ☆ ☆ ☆ ☆

# Strain

Grower _____  Date _____

Acquired _____  $ _____

| Indica | Hybrid | Sativa |

☐ Flower  ☐ Edible  ☐ Concentrate

Sweet / Fruity / Floral / Sour / Spicy / Earthy / Woodsy / Herbal

**Symptoms Relieved**

_____
_____
_____
_____
_____

**Notes**

_____
_____
_____
_____
_____

| Effects | Strength | | | | |
|---|---|---|---|---|---|
| Peaceful | ○ | ○ | ○ | ○ | ○ |
| Sleepy | ○ | ○ | ○ | ○ | ○ |
| Pain Relief | ○ | ○ | ○ | ○ | ○ |
| Hungry | ○ | ○ | ○ | ○ | ○ |
| Uplifted | ○ | ○ | ○ | ○ | ○ |
| Creative | ○ | ○ | ○ | ○ | ○ |

**Ratings** ☆ ☆ ☆ ☆ ☆

# Strain

Grower _____   Date _____

Acquired _____   $ _____

| Indica | Hybrid | Sativa |

☐ Flower   ☐ Edible   ☐ Concentrate

**Symptoms Relieved**
_____
_____
_____
_____

Sweet / Fruity / Floral / Sour / Spicy / Earthy / Herbal / Woodsy

**Notes**
_____
_____
_____
_____
_____

| Effects | Strength | | | | |
|---|---|---|---|---|---|
| Peaceful | ○ | ○ | ○ | ○ | ○ |
| Sleepy | ○ | ○ | ○ | ○ | ○ |
| Pain Relief | ○ | ○ | ○ | ○ | ○ |
| Hungry | ○ | ○ | ○ | ○ | ○ |
| Uplifted | ○ | ○ | ○ | ○ | ○ |
| Creative | ○ | ○ | ○ | ○ | ○ |

**Ratings** ☆ ☆ ☆ ☆ ☆

# Strain

Grower _____  Date _____

Acquired _____  $ _____

| Indica | Hybrid | Sativa |

☐ Flower  ☐ Edible  ☐ Concentrate

**Symptoms Relieved**

_____
_____
_____
_____
_____

Sweet / Fruity / Floral / Spicy / Herbal / Woodsy / Earthy / Sour

**Notes**

_____
_____
_____
_____
_____

| Effects | Strength | | | | |
|---|---|---|---|---|---|
| Peaceful | ○ | ○ | ○ | ○ | ○ |
| Sleepy | ○ | ○ | ○ | ○ | ○ |
| Pain Relief | ○ | ○ | ○ | ○ | ○ |
| Hungry | ○ | ○ | ○ | ○ | ○ |
| Uplifted | ○ | ○ | ○ | ○ | ○ |
| Creative | ○ | ○ | ○ | ○ | ○ |

**Ratings** ☆ ☆ ☆ ☆ ☆

# Strain

Grower _____    Date _____

Acquired _____    $ _____

| Indica | Hybrid | Sativa |

☐ Flower   ☐ Edible   ☐ Concentrate

Sweet
Fruity       Floral
Sour         Spicy
Earthy       Herbal
Woodsy

## Symptoms Relieved

_____
_____
_____
_____

## Notes

_____
_____
_____
_____
_____

| Effects | Strength |
|---|---|
| Peaceful | ○ ○ ○ ○ ○ |
| Sleepy | ○ ○ ○ ○ ○ |
| Pain Relief | ○ ○ ○ ○ ○ |
| Hungry | ○ ○ ○ ○ ○ |
| Uplifted | ○ ○ ○ ○ ○ |
| Creative | ○ ○ ○ ○ ○ |

**Ratings** ☆ ☆ ☆ ☆ ☆

# Strain

Grower _____  Date _____

Acquired _____  $ _____

Indica          Hybrid          Sativa

☐ Flower    ☐ Edible    ☐ Concentrate

**Symptoms Relieved**

_____
_____
_____
_____

Sweet  Fruity  Floral  Sour  Spicy  Earthy  Herbal  Woodsy

**Notes**

_____
_____
_____
_____
_____
_____

| Effects | Strength | | | | |
|---|---|---|---|---|---|
| Peaceful | ○ | ○ | ○ | ○ | ○ |
| Sleepy | ○ | ○ | ○ | ○ | ○ |
| Pain Relief | ○ | ○ | ○ | ○ | ○ |
| Hungry | ○ | ○ | ○ | ○ | ○ |
| Uplifted | ○ | ○ | ○ | ○ | ○ |
| Creative | ○ | ○ | ○ | ○ | ○ |

**Ratings** ☆ ☆ ☆ ☆ ☆

# Strain

Grower _____  Date _____

Acquired _____  $ _____

| Indica | Hybrid | Sativa |

☐ Flower   ☐ Edible   ☐ Concentrate

**Symptoms Relieved**

_____
_____
_____
_____

Sweet · Floral · Spicy · Herbal · Woodsy · Earthy · Sour · Fruity

**Notes**

_____
_____
_____
_____
_____
_____

| Effects | Strength | | | | |
|---|---|---|---|---|---|
| Peaceful | ○ | ○ | ○ | ○ | ○ |
| Sleepy | ○ | ○ | ○ | ○ | ○ |
| Pain Relief | ○ | ○ | ○ | ○ | ○ |
| Hungry | ○ | ○ | ○ | ○ | ○ |
| Uplifted | ○ | ○ | ○ | ○ | ○ |
| Creative | ○ | ○ | ○ | ○ | ○ |

**Ratings** ☆ ☆ ☆ ☆ ☆

# Strain

Grower _____  Date _____

Acquired _____  $ _____

| Indica | Hybrid | Sativa |

☐ Flower  ☐ Edible  ☐ Concentrate

**Symptoms Relieved**

_____
_____
_____
_____
_____

Sweet · Fruity · Floral · Sour · Spicy · Earthy · Woodsy · Herbal

**Notes**

_____
_____
_____
_____
_____
_____

| Effects | Strength | | | | |
|---|---|---|---|---|---|
| Peaceful | ○ | ○ | ○ | ○ | ○ |
| Sleepy | ○ | ○ | ○ | ○ | ○ |
| Pain Relief | ○ | ○ | ○ | ○ | ○ |
| Hungry | ○ | ○ | ○ | ○ | ○ |
| Uplifted | ○ | ○ | ○ | ○ | ○ |
| Creative | ○ | ○ | ○ | ○ | ○ |

**Ratings** ☆ ☆ ☆ ☆ ☆

# Strain

Grower _____  Date _____

Acquired _____  $ _____

Indica          Hybrid          Sativa

☐ Flower   ☐ Edible   ☐ Concentrate

**Symptoms Relieved**

_____
_____
_____
_____
_____

Sweet
Fruity     Floral
Sour     Spicy
Earthy   Herbal
Woodsy

**Notes**

_____
_____
_____
_____
_____
_____

| Effects | Strength | | | | |
|---|---|---|---|---|---|
| Peaceful | ○ | ○ | ○ | ○ | ○ |
| Sleepy | ○ | ○ | ○ | ○ | ○ |
| Pain Relief | ○ | ○ | ○ | ○ | ○ |
| Hungry | ○ | ○ | ○ | ○ | ○ |
| Uplifted | ○ | ○ | ○ | ○ | ○ |
| Creative | ○ | ○ | ○ | ○ | ○ |

**Ratings** ☆ ☆ ☆ ☆ ☆

# Strain

Grower _____  Date _____

Acquired _____  $ _____

| Indica | Hybrid | Sativa |

☐ Flower  ☐ Edible  ☐ Concentrate

**Symptoms Relieved**

_____
_____
_____
_____

Flavor wheel: Sweet, Floral, Spicy, Herbal, Woodsy, Earthy, Sour, Fruity

**Notes**

_____
_____
_____
_____
_____
_____

| Effects | Strength |
|---|---|
| Peaceful | ○ ○ ○ ○ ○ |
| Sleepy | ○ ○ ○ ○ ○ |
| Pain Relief | ○ ○ ○ ○ ○ |
| Hungry | ○ ○ ○ ○ ○ |
| Uplifted | ○ ○ ○ ○ ○ |
| Creative | ○ ○ ○ ○ ○ |

**Ratings** ☆ ☆ ☆ ☆ ☆

# Strain

Grower _____  Date _____

Acquired _____  $ _____

| Indica | Hybrid | Sativa |

☐ Flower  ☐ Edible  ☐ Concentrate

**Symptoms Relieved**

_____
_____
_____
_____
_____

Sweet · Floral · Spicy · Herbal · Woodsy · Earthy · Sour · Fruity

**Notes**

_____
_____
_____
_____
_____
_____

| Effects | Strength |
|---|---|
| Peaceful | ○ ○ ○ ○ ○ |
| Sleepy | ○ ○ ○ ○ ○ |
| Pain Relief | ○ ○ ○ ○ ○ |
| Hungry | ○ ○ ○ ○ ○ |
| Uplifted | ○ ○ ○ ○ ○ |
| Creative | ○ ○ ○ ○ ○ |

**Ratings** ☆ ☆ ☆ ☆ ☆

# Strain

Grower _____   Date _____

Acquired _____   $ _____

| Indica | Hybrid | Sativa |

☐ Flower   ☐ Edible   ☐ Concentrate

**Symptoms Relieved**

_____
_____
_____
_____

Flavor wheel: Sweet, Floral, Spicy, Herbal, Woodsy, Earthy, Sour, Fruity

**Notes**

_____
_____
_____
_____
_____
_____

| Effects | Strength |
|---|---|
| Peaceful | ○ ○ ○ ○ ○ |
| Sleepy | ○ ○ ○ ○ ○ |
| Pain Relief | ○ ○ ○ ○ ○ |
| Hungry | ○ ○ ○ ○ ○ |
| Uplifted | ○ ○ ○ ○ ○ |
| Creative | ○ ○ ○ ○ ○ |

**Ratings** ☆ ☆ ☆ ☆ ☆

# Strain

Grower _____ Date _____

Acquired _____ $ _____

| Indica | Hybrid | Sativa |

☐ Flower  ☐ Edible  ☐ Concentrate

**Symptoms Relieved**
_____
_____
_____
_____
_____

Sweet / Floral / Spicy / Herbal / Woodsy / Earthy / Sour / Fruity

**Notes**
_____
_____
_____
_____
_____

| Effects | Strength | | | | |
|---|---|---|---|---|---|
| Peaceful | ○ | ○ | ○ | ○ | ○ |
| Sleepy | ○ | ○ | ○ | ○ | ○ |
| Pain Relief | ○ | ○ | ○ | ○ | ○ |
| Hungry | ○ | ○ | ○ | ○ | ○ |
| Uplifted | ○ | ○ | ○ | ○ | ○ |
| Creative | ○ | ○ | ○ | ○ | ○ |

**Ratings** ☆ ☆ ☆ ☆ ☆

# Strain

Grower _____    Date _____

Acquired _____    $ _____

| Indica | Hybrid | Sativa |

☐ Flower   ☐ Edible   ☐ Concentrate

Sweet
Fruity    Floral
Sour    Spicy
Earthy    Herbal
Woodsy

**Symptoms Relieved**

_____
_____
_____
_____
_____

**Notes**

_____
_____
_____
_____
_____
_____

| Effects | Strength |
|---|---|
| Peaceful | ○ ○ ○ ○ ○ |
| Sleepy | ○ ○ ○ ○ ○ |
| Pain Relief | ○ ○ ○ ○ ○ |
| Hungry | ○ ○ ○ ○ ○ |
| Uplifted | ○ ○ ○ ○ ○ |
| Creative | ○ ○ ○ ○ ○ |

**Ratings** ☆ ☆ ☆ ☆ ☆

# Strain

Grower _____    Date _____

Acquired _____    $ _____

Indica                Hybrid                Sativa

☐ Flower   ☐ Edible   ☐ Concentrate

Sweet
Fruity        Floral
Sour          Spicy
Earthy        Herbal
Woodsy

**Symptoms Relieved**

_____
_____
_____
_____
_____

**Notes**

_____
_____
_____
_____
_____
_____

| Effects | Strength | | | | |
|---|---|---|---|---|---|
| Peaceful | ○ | ○ | ○ | ○ | ○ |
| Sleepy | ○ | ○ | ○ | ○ | ○ |
| Pain Relief | ○ | ○ | ○ | ○ | ○ |
| Hungry | ○ | ○ | ○ | ○ | ○ |
| Uplifted | ○ | ○ | ○ | ○ | ○ |
| Creative | ○ | ○ | ○ | ○ | ○ |

**Ratings** ☆ ☆ ☆ ☆ ☆

# Strain

Grower _____    Date _____

Acquired _____    $ _____

|  Indica          Hybrid          Sativa  |

☐ Flower   ☐ Edible   ☐ Concentrate

**Symptoms Relieved**

_____
_____
_____
_____
_____

Sweet · Fruity · Floral · Sour · Spicy · Earthy · Herbal · Woodsy

**Notes**

_____
_____
_____
_____
_____
_____

| Effects | Strength |
|---|---|
| Peaceful | ○ ○ ○ ○ ○ |
| Sleepy | ○ ○ ○ ○ ○ |
| Pain Relief | ○ ○ ○ ○ ○ |
| Hungry | ○ ○ ○ ○ ○ |
| Uplifted | ○ ○ ○ ○ ○ |
| Creative | ○ ○ ○ ○ ○ |

**Ratings** ☆ ☆ ☆ ☆ ☆

# Strain

Grower _____  Date _____

Acquired _____  $ _____

| Indica | Hybrid | Sativa |

☐ Flower  ☐ Edible  ☐ Concentrate

```
           Sweet
   Fruity        Floral


Sour                    Spicy


   Earthy        Herbal
           Woodsy
```

**Symptoms Relieved**

_____
_____
_____
_____
_____

**Notes**

_____
_____
_____
_____
_____
_____

| Effects | Strength | | | | |
|---|---|---|---|---|---|
| Peaceful | ○ | ○ | ○ | ○ | ○ |
| Sleepy | ○ | ○ | ○ | ○ | ○ |
| Pain Relief | ○ | ○ | ○ | ○ | ○ |
| Hungry | ○ | ○ | ○ | ○ | ○ |
| Uplifted | ○ | ○ | ○ | ○ | ○ |
| Creative | ○ | ○ | ○ | ○ | ○ |

**Ratings** ☆ ☆ ☆ ☆ ☆

# Strain

Grower _____  Date _____

Acquired _____  $ _____

| Indica | Hybrid | Sativa |

☐ Flower  ☐ Edible  ☐ Concentrate

**Symptoms Relieved**

_____
_____
_____
_____

Sweet
Fruity        Floral
Sour          Spicy
Earthy        Herbal
Woodsy

**Notes**

_____
_____
_____
_____
_____

| Effects | Strength | | | | |
|---|---|---|---|---|---|
| Peaceful | ○ | ○ | ○ | ○ | ○ |
| Sleepy | ○ | ○ | ○ | ○ | ○ |
| Pain Relief | ○ | ○ | ○ | ○ | ○ |
| Hungry | ○ | ○ | ○ | ○ | ○ |
| Uplifted | ○ | ○ | ○ | ○ | ○ |
| Creative | ○ | ○ | ○ | ○ | ○ |

**Ratings** ☆ ☆ ☆ ☆ ☆

# Strain

Grower _____  Date _____

Acquired _____  $ _____

| Indica | Hybrid | Sativa |

☐ Flower  ☐ Edible  ☐ Concentrate

**Symptoms Relieved**

_____
_____
_____
_____

Flavor wheel: Sweet, Floral, Spicy, Herbal, Woodsy, Earthy, Sour, Fruity

**Notes**

_____
_____
_____
_____
_____

| Effects | Strength |
|---|---|
| Peaceful | ○ ○ ○ ○ ○ |
| Sleepy | ○ ○ ○ ○ ○ |
| Pain Relief | ○ ○ ○ ○ ○ |
| Hungry | ○ ○ ○ ○ ○ |
| Uplifted | ○ ○ ○ ○ ○ |
| Creative | ○ ○ ○ ○ ○ |

**Ratings** ☆ ☆ ☆ ☆ ☆

# Strain

Grower _____  Date _____

Acquired _____  $ _____

| Indica | Hybrid | Sativa |

☐ Flower  ☐ Edible  ☐ Concentrate

Sweet / Floral / Spicy / Herbal / Woodsy / Earthy / Sour / Fruity

**Symptoms Relieved**

_____
_____
_____
_____
_____

**Notes**

_____
_____
_____
_____
_____
_____
_____

**Effects** — **Strength**

Peaceful ○ ○ ○ ○ ○
Sleepy ○ ○ ○ ○ ○
Pain Relief ○ ○ ○ ○ ○
Hungry ○ ○ ○ ○ ○
Uplifted ○ ○ ○ ○ ○
Creative ○ ○ ○ ○ ○

**Ratings** ☆ ☆ ☆ ☆ ☆

# Strain

Grower _____  Date _____

Acquired _____  $ _____

| Indica | Hybrid | Sativa |

☐ Flower  ☐ Edible  ☐ Concentrate

**Symptoms Relieved**
_____
_____
_____
_____
_____

**Notes**
_____
_____
_____
_____
_____

Sweet · Floral · Spicy · Herbal · Woodsy · Earthy · Sour · Fruity

| Effects | Strength |
|---|---|
| Peaceful | ○ ○ ○ ○ ○ |
| Sleepy | ○ ○ ○ ○ ○ |
| Pain Relief | ○ ○ ○ ○ ○ |
| Hungry | ○ ○ ○ ○ ○ |
| Uplifted | ○ ○ ○ ○ ○ |
| Creative | ○ ○ ○ ○ ○ |

Ratings ☆ ☆ ☆ ☆ ☆

# Strain

Grower _____  Date _____

Acquired _____  $ _____

| Indica | Hybrid | Sativa |

☐ Flower  ☐ Edible  ☐ Concentrate

**Symptoms Relieved**

_____
_____
_____
_____

Sweet / Fruity / Floral / Sour / Spicy / Earthy / Woodsy / Herbal

**Notes**

_____
_____
_____
_____
_____
_____

| Effects | Strength | | | | |
|---|---|---|---|---|---|
| Peaceful | ○ | ○ | ○ | ○ | ○ |
| Sleepy | ○ | ○ | ○ | ○ | ○ |
| Pain Relief | ○ | ○ | ○ | ○ | ○ |
| Hungry | ○ | ○ | ○ | ○ | ○ |
| Uplifted | ○ | ○ | ○ | ○ | ○ |
| Creative | ○ | ○ | ○ | ○ | ○ |

**Ratings** ☆ ☆ ☆ ☆ ☆

# Strain

Grower _____  Date _____

Acquired _____  $ _____

| Indica | Hybrid | Sativa |

☐ Flower    ☐ Edible    ☐ Concentrate

**Symptoms Relieved**
_____
_____
_____
_____

Sweet · Floral · Spicy · Herbal · Woodsy · Earthy · Sour · Fruity

**Notes**
_____
_____
_____
_____
_____

| Effects | Strength | | | | |
|---|---|---|---|---|---|
| Peaceful | ○ | ○ | ○ | ○ | ○ |
| Sleepy | ○ | ○ | ○ | ○ | ○ |
| Pain Relief | ○ | ○ | ○ | ○ | ○ |
| Hungry | ○ | ○ | ○ | ○ | ○ |
| Uplifted | ○ | ○ | ○ | ○ | ○ |
| Creative | ○ | ○ | ○ | ○ | ○ |

**Ratings** ☆ ☆ ☆ ☆ ☆

# Strain

Grower _____  Date _____
Acquired _____  $ _____

| Indica | Hybrid | Sativa |

☐ Flower    ☐ Edible    ☐ Concentrate

**Symptoms Relieved**
_____
_____
_____
_____

Sweet · Fruity · Floral · Sour · Spicy · Earthy · Herbal · Woodsy

**Notes**
_____
_____
_____
_____
_____

| Effects | Strength |
|---|---|
| Peaceful | ○ ○ ○ ○ ○ |
| Sleepy | ○ ○ ○ ○ ○ |
| Pain Relief | ○ ○ ○ ○ ○ |
| Hungry | ○ ○ ○ ○ ○ |
| Uplifted | ○ ○ ○ ○ ○ |
| Creative | ○ ○ ○ ○ ○ |

**Ratings** ☆ ☆ ☆ ☆ ☆

# Strain

Grower _____  Date _____

Acquired _____  $ _____

| Indica | Hybrid | Sativa |

☐ Flower    ☐ Edible    ☐ Concentrate

**Symptoms Relieved**
_____
_____
_____
_____
_____

Flavor wheel: Sweet, Floral, Spicy, Herbal, Woodsy, Earthy, Sour, Fruity

**Notes**
_____
_____
_____
_____
_____
_____
_____

| Effects | Strength | | | | |
|---|---|---|---|---|---|
| Peaceful | ○ | ○ | ○ | ○ | ○ |
| Sleepy | ○ | ○ | ○ | ○ | ○ |
| Pain Relief | ○ | ○ | ○ | ○ | ○ |
| Hungry | ○ | ○ | ○ | ○ | ○ |
| Uplifted | ○ | ○ | ○ | ○ | ○ |
| Creative | ○ | ○ | ○ | ○ | ○ |

**Ratings** ☆ ☆ ☆ ☆ ☆

# Strain

Grower _____  Date _____

Acquired _____  $ _____

| Indica | Hybrid | Sativa |

☐ Flower  ☐ Edible  ☐ Concentrate

**Symptoms Relieved**

_____
_____
_____
_____
_____

Flavor wheel: Sweet, Floral, Spicy, Herbal, Woodsy, Earthy, Sour, Fruity

**Notes**

_____
_____
_____
_____
_____
_____

| Effects | Strength | | | | |
|---|---|---|---|---|---|
| Peaceful | ○ | ○ | ○ | ○ | ○ |
| Sleepy | ○ | ○ | ○ | ○ | ○ |
| Pain Relief | ○ | ○ | ○ | ○ | ○ |
| Hungry | ○ | ○ | ○ | ○ | ○ |
| Uplifted | ○ | ○ | ○ | ○ | ○ |
| Creative | ○ | ○ | ○ | ○ | ○ |

**Ratings** ☆ ☆ ☆ ☆ ☆

# Strain

Grower _____  Date _____

Acquired _____  $ _____

| Indica | Hybrid | Sativa |

☐ Flower  ☐ Edible  ☐ Concentrate

Sweet / Fruity / Floral / Sour / Spicy / Earthy / Woodsy / Herbal

**Symptoms Relieved**

_____
_____
_____
_____
_____

**Notes**

_____
_____
_____
_____
_____
_____

| Effects | Strength | | | | |
|---|---|---|---|---|---|
| Peaceful | ○ | ○ | ○ | ○ | ○ |
| Sleepy | ○ | ○ | ○ | ○ | ○ |
| Pain Relief | ○ | ○ | ○ | ○ | ○ |
| Hungry | ○ | ○ | ○ | ○ | ○ |
| Uplifted | ○ | ○ | ○ | ○ | ○ |
| Creative | ○ | ○ | ○ | ○ | ○ |

**Ratings** ☆ ☆ ☆ ☆ ☆

# Strain

Grower _____ Date _____

Acquired _____ $ _____

| Indica | Hybrid | Sativa |

☐ Flower  ☐ Edible  ☐ Concentrate

**Symptoms Relieved**

_____
_____
_____
_____
_____

Sweet • Floral • Spicy • Herbal • Woodsy • Earthy • Sour • Fruity

**Notes**

_____
_____
_____
_____
_____
_____
_____

| Effects | Strength |
|---|---|
| Peaceful | ○ ○ ○ ○ ○ |
| Sleepy | ○ ○ ○ ○ ○ |
| Pain Relief | ○ ○ ○ ○ ○ |
| Hungry | ○ ○ ○ ○ ○ |
| Uplifted | ○ ○ ○ ○ ○ |
| Creative | ○ ○ ○ ○ ○ |

**Ratings** ☆ ☆ ☆ ☆ ☆

# Strain

Grower _____  Date _____

Acquired _____  $ _____

|  Indica          Hybrid          Sativa  |

☐ Flower   ☐ Edible   ☐ Concentrate

```
           Sweet
  Fruity          Floral

Sour                     Spicy

  Earthy          Herbal
          Woodsy
```

**Symptoms Relieved**

_____
_____
_____
_____
_____

**Notes**

_____
_____
_____
_____
_____
_____

| Effects | Strength |
|---|---|
| Peaceful | ○ ○ ○ ○ ○ |
| Sleepy | ○ ○ ○ ○ ○ |
| Pain Relief | ○ ○ ○ ○ ○ |
| Hungry | ○ ○ ○ ○ ○ |
| Uplifted | ○ ○ ○ ○ ○ |
| Creative | ○ ○ ○ ○ ○ |

**Ratings** ☆ ☆ ☆ ☆ ☆

# Strain

Grower _____ Date _____

Acquired _____ $ _____

| Indica | Hybrid | Sativa |

☐ Flower  ☐ Edible  ☐ Concentrate

**Symptoms Relieved**

_____
_____
_____
_____

Sweet · Floral · Spicy · Herbal · Woodsy · Earthy · Sour · Fruity

**Notes**

_____
_____
_____
_____
_____
_____

| Effects | Strength | | | | |
|---|---|---|---|---|---|
| Peaceful | ○ | ○ | ○ | ○ | ○ |
| Sleepy | ○ | ○ | ○ | ○ | ○ |
| Pain Relief | ○ | ○ | ○ | ○ | ○ |
| Hungry | ○ | ○ | ○ | ○ | ○ |
| Uplifted | ○ | ○ | ○ | ○ | ○ |
| Creative | ○ | ○ | ○ | ○ | ○ |

**Ratings** ☆ ☆ ☆ ☆ ☆

# Strain

Grower _____  Date _____

Acquired _____  $ _____

| Indica | Hybrid | Sativa |

☐ Flower  ☐ Edible  ☐ Concentrate

**Symptoms Relieved**
_____
_____
_____
_____

Sweet
Fruity     Floral
Sour       Spicy
Earthy     Herbal
Woodsy

**Notes**
_____
_____
_____
_____
_____
_____

| Effects | Strength |
|---|---|
| Peaceful | ○ ○ ○ ○ ○ |
| Sleepy | ○ ○ ○ ○ ○ |
| Pain Relief | ○ ○ ○ ○ ○ |
| Hungry | ○ ○ ○ ○ ○ |
| Uplifted | ○ ○ ○ ○ ○ |
| Creative | ○ ○ ○ ○ ○ |

**Ratings** ☆ ☆ ☆ ☆ ☆

# Strain

Grower _____   Date _____

Acquired _____   $ _____

| Indica | Hybrid | Sativa |

☐ Flower   ☐ Edible   ☐ Concentrate

**Symptoms Relieved**

_____
_____
_____
_____
_____

Sweet · Fruity · Floral · Sour · Spicy · Earthy · Woodsy · Herbal

**Notes**

_____
_____
_____
_____
_____
_____
_____

| Effects | Strength | | | | |
|---|---|---|---|---|---|
| Peaceful | ○ | ○ | ○ | ○ | ○ |
| Sleepy | ○ | ○ | ○ | ○ | ○ |
| Pain Relief | ○ | ○ | ○ | ○ | ○ |
| Hungry | ○ | ○ | ○ | ○ | ○ |
| Uplifted | ○ | ○ | ○ | ○ | ○ |
| Creative | ○ | ○ | ○ | ○ | ○ |

**Ratings** ☆ ☆ ☆ ☆ ☆

# Strain

Grower _____ Date _____

Acquired _____ $ _____

| Indica | Hybrid | Sativa |

☐ Flower  ☐ Edible  ☐ Concentrate

**Symptoms Relieved**

_____
_____
_____
_____
_____

Sweet · Floral · Spicy · Herbal · Woodsy · Earthy · Sour · Fruity

**Notes**

_____
_____
_____
_____
_____
_____

| Effects | Strength | | | | |
|---|---|---|---|---|---|
| Peaceful | ○ | ○ | ○ | ○ | ○ |
| Sleepy | ○ | ○ | ○ | ○ | ○ |
| Pain Relief | ○ | ○ | ○ | ○ | ○ |
| Hungry | ○ | ○ | ○ | ○ | ○ |
| Uplifted | ○ | ○ | ○ | ○ | ○ |
| Creative | ○ | ○ | ○ | ○ | ○ |

**Ratings** ☆ ☆ ☆ ☆ ☆

# Strain

Grower _____  Date _____

Acquired _____  $ _____

| Indica | Hybrid | Sativa |

☐ Flower  ☐ Edible  ☐ Concentrate

**Symptoms Relieved**

_____
_____
_____
_____

Sweet · Fruity · Floral · Sour · Spicy · Earthy · Woodsy · Herbal

**Notes**

_____
_____
_____
_____
_____
_____

| Effects | Strength | | | | |
|---|---|---|---|---|---|
| Peaceful | ○ | ○ | ○ | ○ | ○ |
| Sleepy | ○ | ○ | ○ | ○ | ○ |
| Pain Relief | ○ | ○ | ○ | ○ | ○ |
| Hungry | ○ | ○ | ○ | ○ | ○ |
| Uplifted | ○ | ○ | ○ | ○ | ○ |
| Creative | ○ | ○ | ○ | ○ | ○ |

**Ratings** ☆ ☆ ☆ ☆ ☆

# Strain

Grower _____    Date _____

Acquired _____    $ _____

Indica          Hybrid          Sativa

☐ Flower   ☐ Edible   ☐ Concentrate

## Symptoms Relieved

_____
_____
_____
_____

Sweet  
Fruity   Floral  
Sour   Spicy  
Earthy   Herbal  
Woodsy

## Notes

_____
_____
_____
_____
_____
_____

| Effects | Strength | | | | |
|---|---|---|---|---|---|
| Peaceful | ○ | ○ | ○ | ○ | ○ |
| Sleepy | ○ | ○ | ○ | ○ | ○ |
| Pain Relief | ○ | ○ | ○ | ○ | ○ |
| Hungry | ○ | ○ | ○ | ○ | ○ |
| Uplifted | ○ | ○ | ○ | ○ | ○ |
| Creative | ○ | ○ | ○ | ○ | ○ |

**Ratings** ☆ ☆ ☆ ☆ ☆

# Strain

Grower _____    Date _____

Acquired _____    $ _____

| Indica | Hybrid | Sativa |

☐ Flower   ☐ Edible   ☐ Concentrate

**Symptoms Relieved**

_____
_____
_____
_____

Sweet · Floral · Spicy · Herbal · Woodsy · Earthy · Sour · Fruity

**Notes**

_____
_____
_____
_____
_____
_____

| Effects | Strength | | | | |
|---|---|---|---|---|---|
| Peaceful | ○ | ○ | ○ | ○ | ○ |
| Sleepy | ○ | ○ | ○ | ○ | ○ |
| Pain Relief | ○ | ○ | ○ | ○ | ○ |
| Hungry | ○ | ○ | ○ | ○ | ○ |
| Uplifted | ○ | ○ | ○ | ○ | ○ |
| Creative | ○ | ○ | ○ | ○ | ○ |

**Ratings** ☆ ☆ ☆ ☆ ☆

# Strain

Grower _____   Date _____

Acquired _____   $ _____

|  Indica | Hybrid | Sativa |

☐ Flower   ☐ Edible   ☐ Concentrate

**Symptoms Relieved**

_____
_____
_____
_____
_____

Sweet · Floral · Spicy · Herbal · Woodsy · Earthy · Sour · Fruity

**Notes**

_____
_____
_____
_____
_____

| Effects | Strength | | | | |
|---|---|---|---|---|---|
| Peaceful | ○ | ○ | ○ | ○ | ○ |
| Sleepy | ○ | ○ | ○ | ○ | ○ |
| Pain Relief | ○ | ○ | ○ | ○ | ○ |
| Hungry | ○ | ○ | ○ | ○ | ○ |
| Uplifted | ○ | ○ | ○ | ○ | ○ |
| Creative | ○ | ○ | ○ | ○ | ○ |

**Ratings** ☆ ☆ ☆ ☆ ☆

# Strain

Grower _____   Date _____

Acquired _____   $ _____

---

Indica          Hybrid          Sativa

---

☐ Flower   ☐ Edible   ☐ Concentrate

**Symptoms Relieved**

_____
_____
_____
_____

Sweet · Floral · Spicy · Herbal · Woodsy · Earthy · Sour · Fruity

**Notes**

_____
_____
_____
_____
_____

| Effects | Strength | | | | |
|---|---|---|---|---|---|
| Peaceful | ○ | ○ | ○ | ○ | ○ |
| Sleepy | ○ | ○ | ○ | ○ | ○ |
| Pain Relief | ○ | ○ | ○ | ○ | ○ |
| Hungry | ○ | ○ | ○ | ○ | ○ |
| Uplifted | ○ | ○ | ○ | ○ | ○ |
| Creative | ○ | ○ | ○ | ○ | ○ |

**Ratings** ☆ ☆ ☆ ☆ ☆

# Strain

Grower _____  Date _____

Acquired _____  $ _____

| Indica | Hybrid | Sativa |

☐ Flower   ☐ Edible   ☐ Concentrate

**Symptoms Relieved**

_____
_____
_____
_____

Sweet · Floral · Spicy · Herbal · Woodsy · Earthy · Sour · Fruity

**Notes**

_____
_____
_____
_____
_____
_____

| Effects | Strength | | | | |
|---|---|---|---|---|---|
| Peaceful | ○ | ○ | ○ | ○ | ○ |
| Sleepy | ○ | ○ | ○ | ○ | ○ |
| Pain Relief | ○ | ○ | ○ | ○ | ○ |
| Hungry | ○ | ○ | ○ | ○ | ○ |
| Uplifted | ○ | ○ | ○ | ○ | ○ |
| Creative | ○ | ○ | ○ | ○ | ○ |

**Ratings** ☆ ☆ ☆ ☆ ☆

# Strain

Grower _____  Date _____

Acquired _____  $ _____

| Indica | Hybrid | Sativa |

☐ Flower    ☐ Edible    ☐ Concentrate

**Symptoms Relieved**

_____
_____
_____
_____
_____

Sweet · Floral · Spicy · Herbal · Woodsy · Earthy · Sour · Fruity

**Notes**

_____
_____
_____
_____
_____
_____
_____

| Effects | Strength |
|---|---|
| Peaceful | ○ ○ ○ ○ ○ |
| Sleepy | ○ ○ ○ ○ ○ |
| Pain Relief | ○ ○ ○ ○ ○ |
| Hungry | ○ ○ ○ ○ ○ |
| Uplifted | ○ ○ ○ ○ ○ |
| Creative | ○ ○ ○ ○ ○ |

**Ratings** ☆ ☆ ☆ ☆ ☆

# Strain

Grower _____  Date _____

Acquired _____  $ _____

| Indica | Hybrid | Sativa |

☐ Flower   ☐ Edible   ☐ Concentrate

**Symptoms Relieved**

_____
_____
_____
_____
_____

Flavor wheel: Sweet, Floral, Spicy, Herbal, Woodsy, Earthy, Sour, Fruity

**Notes**

_____
_____
_____
_____
_____
_____
_____

| Effects | Strength | | | | |
|---|---|---|---|---|---|
| Peaceful | ○ | ○ | ○ | ○ | ○ |
| Sleepy | ○ | ○ | ○ | ○ | ○ |
| Pain Relief | ○ | ○ | ○ | ○ | ○ |
| Hungry | ○ | ○ | ○ | ○ | ○ |
| Uplifted | ○ | ○ | ○ | ○ | ○ |
| Creative | ○ | ○ | ○ | ○ | ○ |

**Ratings** ☆ ☆ ☆ ☆ ☆

# Strain

Grower _____  Date _____

Acquired _____  $ _____

| Indica | Hybrid | Sativa |

☐ Flower  ☐ Edible  ☐ Concentrate

**Symptoms Relieved**

_____
_____
_____
_____

Sweet · Fruity · Floral · Sour · Spicy · Earthy · Herbal · Woodsy

**Notes**

_____
_____
_____
_____
_____
_____

| Effects | Strength | | | | |
|---|---|---|---|---|---|
| Peaceful | ○ | ○ | ○ | ○ | ○ |
| Sleepy | ○ | ○ | ○ | ○ | ○ |
| Pain Relief | ○ | ○ | ○ | ○ | ○ |
| Hungry | ○ | ○ | ○ | ○ | ○ |
| Uplifted | ○ | ○ | ○ | ○ | ○ |
| Creative | ○ | ○ | ○ | ○ | ○ |

**Ratings** ☆ ☆ ☆ ☆ ☆

# Strain

Grower _____  Date _____

Acquired _____  $ _____

Indica          Hybrid          Sativa

☐ Flower   ☐ Edible   ☐ Concentrate

**Symptoms Relieved**
_____
_____
_____
_____

Sweet, Fruity, Floral, Sour, Spicy, Earthy, Woodsy, Herbal

**Notes**
_____
_____
_____
_____
_____

| Effects | Strength | | | | |
|---|---|---|---|---|---|
| Peaceful | ○ | ○ | ○ | ○ | ○ |
| Sleepy | ○ | ○ | ○ | ○ | ○ |
| Pain Relief | ○ | ○ | ○ | ○ | ○ |
| Hungry | ○ | ○ | ○ | ○ | ○ |
| Uplifted | ○ | ○ | ○ | ○ | ○ |
| Creative | ○ | ○ | ○ | ○ | ○ |

**Ratings** ☆ ☆ ☆ ☆ ☆

# Strain

Grower _____   Date _____

Acquired _____   $ _____

|  Indica  |  Hybrid  |  Sativa  |

☐ Flower   ☐ Edible   ☐ Concentrate

**Symptoms Relieved**

_____
_____
_____
_____

Sweet · Fruity · Floral · Sour · Spicy · Earthy · Herbal · Woodsy

**Notes**

_____
_____
_____
_____
_____

| Effects | Strength | | | | |
|---|---|---|---|---|---|
| Peaceful | ○ | ○ | ○ | ○ | ○ |
| Sleepy | ○ | ○ | ○ | ○ | ○ |
| Pain Relief | ○ | ○ | ○ | ○ | ○ |
| Hungry | ○ | ○ | ○ | ○ | ○ |
| Uplifted | ○ | ○ | ○ | ○ | ○ |
| Creative | ○ | ○ | ○ | ○ | ○ |

**Ratings** ☆ ☆ ☆ ☆ ☆

# Strain

Grower _____  Date _____

Acquired _____  $ _____

Indica                Hybrid                Sativa

☐ Flower   ☐ Edible   ☐ Concentrate

Sweet
Fruity          Floral
Sour            Spicy
Earthy          Herbal
Woodsy

**Symptoms Relieved**

_____
_____
_____
_____

**Notes**

_____
_____
_____
_____
_____
_____

| Effects | Strength | | | | |
|---|---|---|---|---|---|
| Peaceful | ○ | ○ | ○ | ○ | ○ |
| Sleepy | ○ | ○ | ○ | ○ | ○ |
| Pain Relief | ○ | ○ | ○ | ○ | ○ |
| Hungry | ○ | ○ | ○ | ○ | ○ |
| Uplifted | ○ | ○ | ○ | ○ | ○ |
| Creative | ○ | ○ | ○ | ○ | ○ |

**Ratings** ☆ ☆ ☆ ☆ ☆

# Strain

Grower _____  Date _____

Acquired _____  $ _____

| Indica | Hybrid | Sativa |

☐ Flower   ☐ Edible   ☐ Concentrate

**Symptoms Relieved**
_____
_____
_____
_____
_____

Sweet, Fruity, Floral, Sour, Spicy, Earthy, Woodsy, Herbal

**Notes**
_____
_____
_____
_____
_____
_____
_____

| Effects | Strength |
|---|---|
| Peaceful | ○ ○ ○ ○ ○ |
| Sleepy | ○ ○ ○ ○ ○ |
| Pain Relief | ○ ○ ○ ○ ○ |
| Hungry | ○ ○ ○ ○ ○ |
| Uplifted | ○ ○ ○ ○ ○ |
| Creative | ○ ○ ○ ○ ○ |

**Ratings** ☆ ☆ ☆ ☆ ☆

# Strain

Grower _____    Date _____

Acquired _____    $ _____

| Indica | Hybrid | Sativa |

☐ Flower  ☐ Edible  ☐ Concentrate

**Symptoms Relieved**

_____
_____
_____
_____
_____

Sweet · Floral · Spicy · Herbal · Woodsy · Earthy · Sour · Fruity

**Notes**

_____
_____
_____
_____
_____
_____
_____

| Effects | Strength | | | | |
|---|---|---|---|---|---|
| Peaceful | ○ | ○ | ○ | ○ | ○ |
| Sleepy | ○ | ○ | ○ | ○ | ○ |
| Pain Relief | ○ | ○ | ○ | ○ | ○ |
| Hungry | ○ | ○ | ○ | ○ | ○ |
| Uplifted | ○ | ○ | ○ | ○ | ○ |
| Creative | ○ | ○ | ○ | ○ | ○ |

**Ratings** ☆ ☆ ☆ ☆ ☆

# Strain

Grower _____  Date _____

Acquired _____  $ _____

|     Indica     |     Hybrid     |     Sativa     |

☐ Flower    ☐ Edible    ☐ Concentrate

**Symptoms Relieved**

_____
_____
_____
_____
_____

Flavor wheel: Sweet, Floral, Spicy, Herbal, Woodsy, Earthy, Sour, Fruity

**Notes**

_____
_____
_____
_____
_____
_____
_____

| Effects | Strength |
|---|---|
| Peaceful | ○ ○ ○ ○ ○ |
| Sleepy | ○ ○ ○ ○ ○ |
| Pain Relief | ○ ○ ○ ○ ○ |
| Hungry | ○ ○ ○ ○ ○ |
| Uplifted | ○ ○ ○ ○ ○ |
| Creative | ○ ○ ○ ○ ○ |

**Ratings** ☆ ☆ ☆ ☆ ☆

# Strain

Grower _____ Date _____

Acquired _____ $ _____

| Indica | Hybrid | Sativa |

☐ Flower  ☐ Edible  ☐ Concentrate

Sweet
Fruity        Floral

**Symptoms Relieved**

Sour                    Spicy

_____
_____
_____
_____
_____

Earthy         Herbal
Woodsy

| Effects | Strength |
| --- | --- |
| Peaceful | ○ ○ ○ ○ ○ |
| Sleepy | ○ ○ ○ ○ ○ |
| Pain Relief | ○ ○ ○ ○ ○ |
| Hungry | ○ ○ ○ ○ ○ |
| Uplifted | ○ ○ ○ ○ ○ |
| Creative | ○ ○ ○ ○ ○ |

**Notes**

_____
_____
_____
_____
_____
_____

**Ratings** ☆ ☆ ☆ ☆ ☆

# Strain

Grower _____  Date _____

Acquired _____  $ _____

| Indica | Hybrid | Sativa |

☐ Flower  ☐ Edible  ☐ Concentrate

**Symptoms Relieved**

_____
_____
_____
_____

Sweet / Floral / Spicy / Herbal / Woodsy / Earthy / Sour / Fruity

**Notes**

_____
_____
_____
_____
_____

| Effects | Strength | | | | |
|---|---|---|---|---|---|
| Peaceful | ○ | ○ | ○ | ○ | ○ |
| Sleepy | ○ | ○ | ○ | ○ | ○ |
| Pain Relief | ○ | ○ | ○ | ○ | ○ |
| Hungry | ○ | ○ | ○ | ○ | ○ |
| Uplifted | ○ | ○ | ○ | ○ | ○ |
| Creative | ○ | ○ | ○ | ○ | ○ |

**Ratings** ☆ ☆ ☆ ☆ ☆

# Strain

Grower _____  Date _____

Acquired _____  $ _____

| Indica | Hybrid | Sativa |

☐ Flower  ☐ Edible  ☐ Concentrate

**Symptoms Relieved**

_____
_____
_____
_____

Flavor wheel: Sweet, Floral, Spicy, Herbal, Woodsy, Earthy, Sour, Fruity

**Notes**

_____
_____
_____
_____
_____

| Effects | Strength | | | | |
|---|---|---|---|---|---|
| Peaceful | ○ | ○ | ○ | ○ | ○ |
| Sleepy | ○ | ○ | ○ | ○ | ○ |
| Pain Relief | ○ | ○ | ○ | ○ | ○ |
| Hungry | ○ | ○ | ○ | ○ | ○ |
| Uplifted | ○ | ○ | ○ | ○ | ○ |
| Creative | ○ | ○ | ○ | ○ | ○ |

**Ratings** ☆ ☆ ☆ ☆ ☆

# Strain

Grower _____  Date _____

Acquired _____  $ _____

| Indica | Hybrid | Sativa |

☐ Flower   ☐ Edible   ☐ Concentrate

**Symptoms Relieved**

_____
_____
_____
_____
_____

Sweet · Fruity · Floral · Sour · Spicy · Earthy · Woodsy · Herbal

**Notes**

_____
_____
_____
_____
_____
_____

| Effects | Strength | | | | |
|---|---|---|---|---|---|
| Peaceful | ○ | ○ | ○ | ○ | ○ |
| Sleepy | ○ | ○ | ○ | ○ | ○ |
| Pain Relief | ○ | ○ | ○ | ○ | ○ |
| Hungry | ○ | ○ | ○ | ○ | ○ |
| Uplifted | ○ | ○ | ○ | ○ | ○ |
| Creative | ○ | ○ | ○ | ○ | ○ |

**Ratings** ☆ ☆ ☆ ☆ ☆

# Strain

Grower _____  Date _____

Acquired _____  $ _____

| Indica | Hybrid | Sativa |

☐ Flower  ☐ Edible  ☐ Concentrate

**Symptoms Relieved**

_____
_____
_____
_____

Sweet
Fruity    Floral
Sour        Spicy
Earthy    Herbal
Woodsy

**Notes**

_____
_____
_____
_____
_____

| Effects | Strength | | | | |
|---|---|---|---|---|---|
| Peaceful | ○ | ○ | ○ | ○ | ○ |
| Sleepy | ○ | ○ | ○ | ○ | ○ |
| Pain Relief | ○ | ○ | ○ | ○ | ○ |
| Hungry | ○ | ○ | ○ | ○ | ○ |
| Uplifted | ○ | ○ | ○ | ○ | ○ |
| Creative | ○ | ○ | ○ | ○ | ○ |

**Ratings** ☆ ☆ ☆ ☆ ☆

# Strain

Grower _____   Date _____

Acquired _____   $ _____

Indica          Hybrid          Sativa

☐ Flower   ☐ Edible   ☐ Concentrate

Sweet
Fruity          Floral
Sour            Spicy
Earthy          Herbal
Woodsy

## Symptoms Relieved

_____
_____
_____
_____

## Notes

_____
_____
_____
_____
_____
_____

| Effects | Strength |
|---|---|
| Peaceful | ○ ○ ○ ○ ○ |
| Sleepy | ○ ○ ○ ○ ○ |
| Pain Relief | ○ ○ ○ ○ ○ |
| Hungry | ○ ○ ○ ○ ○ |
| Uplifted | ○ ○ ○ ○ ○ |
| Creative | ○ ○ ○ ○ ○ |

**Ratings** ☆ ☆ ☆ ☆ ☆

# Strain

Grower _____    Date _____

Acquired _____    $ _____

| Indica | Hybrid | Sativa |

☐ Flower    ☐ Edible    ☐ Concentrate

**Symptoms Relieved**

_____
_____
_____
_____
_____

Sweet · Floral · Spicy · Herbal · Woodsy · Earthy · Sour · Fruity

**Notes**

_____
_____
_____
_____
_____
_____

| Effects | Strength | | | | |
|---|---|---|---|---|---|
| Peaceful | ○ | ○ | ○ | ○ | ○ |
| Sleepy | ○ | ○ | ○ | ○ | ○ |
| Pain Relief | ○ | ○ | ○ | ○ | ○ |
| Hungry | ○ | ○ | ○ | ○ | ○ |
| Uplifted | ○ | ○ | ○ | ○ | ○ |
| Creative | ○ | ○ | ○ | ○ | ○ |

**Ratings** ☆ ☆ ☆ ☆ ☆

# Strain

Grower _____ Date _____

Acquired _____ $ _____

| Indica | Hybrid | Sativa |

☐ Flower  ☐ Edible  ☐ Concentrate

**Symptoms Relieved**

_____
_____
_____
_____

Flavor wheel: Sweet, Floral, Spicy, Herbal, Woodsy, Earthy, Sour, Fruity

**Notes**

_____
_____
_____
_____
_____

| Effects | Strength |
|---|---|
| Peaceful | ○ ○ ○ ○ ○ |
| Sleepy | ○ ○ ○ ○ ○ |
| Pain Relief | ○ ○ ○ ○ ○ |
| Hungry | ○ ○ ○ ○ ○ |
| Uplifted | ○ ○ ○ ○ ○ |
| Creative | ○ ○ ○ ○ ○ |

**Ratings** ☆ ☆ ☆ ☆ ☆

# Strain

Grower _____    Date _____

Acquired _____    $ _____

| Indica | Hybrid | Sativa |

☐ Flower   ☐ Edible   ☐ Concentrate

**Symptoms Relieved**

_____
_____
_____
_____
_____

Flavor wheel: Sweet, Floral, Spicy, Herbal, Woodsy, Earthy, Sour, Fruity

**Notes**

_____
_____
_____
_____
_____
_____

| Effects | Strength | | | | |
|---|---|---|---|---|---|
| Peaceful | ○ | ○ | ○ | ○ | ○ |
| Sleepy | ○ | ○ | ○ | ○ | ○ |
| Pain Relief | ○ | ○ | ○ | ○ | ○ |
| Hungry | ○ | ○ | ○ | ○ | ○ |
| Uplifted | ○ | ○ | ○ | ○ | ○ |
| Creative | ○ | ○ | ○ | ○ | ○ |

**Ratings** ☆ ☆ ☆ ☆ ☆

# Strain

Grower _____  Date _____

Acquired _____  $ _____

| Indica | Hybrid | Sativa |

☐ Flower  ☐ Edible  ☐ Concentrate

**Symptoms Relieved**

_____
_____
_____
_____

Sweet / Fruity / Floral / Sour / Spicy / Earthy / Woodsy / Herbal

**Notes**

_____
_____
_____
_____
_____
_____

| Effects | Strength | | | | |
|---|---|---|---|---|---|
| Peaceful | ○ | ○ | ○ | ○ | ○ |
| Sleepy | ○ | ○ | ○ | ○ | ○ |
| Pain Relief | ○ | ○ | ○ | ○ | ○ |
| Hungry | ○ | ○ | ○ | ○ | ○ |
| Uplifted | ○ | ○ | ○ | ○ | ○ |
| Creative | ○ | ○ | ○ | ○ | ○ |

**Ratings** ☆ ☆ ☆ ☆ ☆

# Strain

Grower _____  Date _____

Acquired _____  $ _____

| Indica | Hybrid | Sativa |

☐ Flower  ☐ Edible  ☐ Concentrate

**Symptoms Relieved**

_____
_____
_____
_____
_____

Flavor wheel: Sweet, Floral, Spicy, Herbal, Woodsy, Earthy, Sour, Fruity

**Notes**

_____
_____
_____
_____
_____
_____

| Effects | Strength | | | | |
|---|---|---|---|---|---|
| Peaceful | ○ | ○ | ○ | ○ | ○ |
| Sleepy | ○ | ○ | ○ | ○ | ○ |
| Pain Relief | ○ | ○ | ○ | ○ | ○ |
| Hungry | ○ | ○ | ○ | ○ | ○ |
| Uplifted | ○ | ○ | ○ | ○ | ○ |
| Creative | ○ | ○ | ○ | ○ | ○ |

**Ratings** ☆ ☆ ☆ ☆ ☆

# Strain

Grower _____ Date _____

Acquired _____ $ _____

| Indica | Hybrid | Sativa |

☐ Flower  ☐ Edible  ☐ Concentrate

**Symptoms Relieved**

_____
_____
_____
_____

Sweet / Floral / Spicy / Herbal / Woodsy / Earthy / Sour / Fruity

**Notes**

_____
_____
_____
_____
_____

| Effects | Strength |
|---|---|
| Peaceful | ○ ○ ○ ○ ○ |
| Sleepy | ○ ○ ○ ○ ○ |
| Pain Relief | ○ ○ ○ ○ ○ |
| Hungry | ○ ○ ○ ○ ○ |
| Uplifted | ○ ○ ○ ○ ○ |
| Creative | ○ ○ ○ ○ ○ |

**Ratings** ☆ ☆ ☆ ☆ ☆

# Strain

Grower _____    Date _____

Acquired _____    $ _____

Indica            Hybrid            Sativa

☐ Flower    ☐ Edible    ☐ Concentrate

Sweet
Fruity        Floral
Sour        Spicy
Earthy        Herbal
Woodsy

**Symptoms Relieved**
_____
_____
_____
_____
_____

**Notes**
_____
_____
_____
_____
_____
_____

| Effects | Strength | | | | |
|---|---|---|---|---|---|
| Peaceful | ○ | ○ | ○ | ○ | ○ |
| Sleepy | ○ | ○ | ○ | ○ | ○ |
| Pain Relief | ○ | ○ | ○ | ○ | ○ |
| Hungry | ○ | ○ | ○ | ○ | ○ |
| Uplifted | ○ | ○ | ○ | ○ | ○ |
| Creative | ○ | ○ | ○ | ○ | ○ |

**Ratings** ☆ ☆ ☆ ☆ ☆

# Strain

Grower _____  Date _____

Acquired _____  $ _____

| Indica | Hybrid | Sativa |

☐ Flower    ☐ Edible    ☐ Concentrate

**Symptoms Relieved**

_____
_____
_____
_____
_____

Sweet / Fruity / Floral / Sour / Spicy / Earthy / Woodsy / Herbal

**Notes**

_____
_____
_____
_____
_____
_____
_____

| Effects | Strength | | | | |
|---|---|---|---|---|---|
| Peaceful | ○ | ○ | ○ | ○ | ○ |
| Sleepy | ○ | ○ | ○ | ○ | ○ |
| Pain Relief | ○ | ○ | ○ | ○ | ○ |
| Hungry | ○ | ○ | ○ | ○ | ○ |
| Uplifted | ○ | ○ | ○ | ○ | ○ |
| Creative | ○ | ○ | ○ | ○ | ○ |

**Ratings** ☆ ☆ ☆ ☆ ☆

# Strain

Grower _____  Date _____

Acquired _____  $ _____

| Indica | Hybrid | Sativa |

☐ Flower  ☐ Edible  ☐ Concentrate

Sweet · Floral · Spicy · Herbal · Woodsy · Earthy · Sour · Fruity

**Symptoms Relieved**
_____
_____
_____
_____
_____

**Notes**
_____
_____
_____
_____
_____
_____

| Effects | Strength |
|---|---|
| Peaceful | ○ ○ ○ ○ ○ |
| Sleepy | ○ ○ ○ ○ ○ |
| Pain Relief | ○ ○ ○ ○ ○ |
| Hungry | ○ ○ ○ ○ ○ |
| Uplifted | ○ ○ ○ ○ ○ |
| Creative | ○ ○ ○ ○ ○ |

**Ratings** ☆ ☆ ☆ ☆ ☆

# Strain

Grower _____   Date _____

Acquired _____   $ _____

| Indica | Hybrid | Sativa |

☐ Flower    ☐ Edible    ☐ Concentrate

**Symptoms Relieved**

_____
_____
_____
_____
_____

Sweet • Floral • Spicy • Herbal • Woodsy • Earthy • Sour • Fruity

**Notes**

_____
_____
_____
_____
_____
_____

| Effects | Strength | | | | |
|---|---|---|---|---|---|
| Peaceful | ○ | ○ | ○ | ○ | ○ |
| Sleepy | ○ | ○ | ○ | ○ | ○ |
| Pain Relief | ○ | ○ | ○ | ○ | ○ |
| Hungry | ○ | ○ | ○ | ○ | ○ |
| Uplifted | ○ | ○ | ○ | ○ | ○ |
| Creative | ○ | ○ | ○ | ○ | ○ |

**Ratings** ☆ ☆ ☆ ☆ ☆

# Strain

Grower _____ Date _____

Acquired _____ $ _____

| Indica | Hybrid | Sativa |

☐ Flower  ☐ Edible  ☐ Concentrate

Sweet / Floral / Spicy / Herbal / Woodsy / Earthy / Sour / Fruity

## Symptoms Relieved

_____
_____
_____
_____

## Notes

_____
_____
_____
_____
_____

| Effects | Strength |
|---|---|
| Peaceful | ○ ○ ○ ○ ○ |
| Sleepy | ○ ○ ○ ○ ○ |
| Pain Relief | ○ ○ ○ ○ ○ |
| Hungry | ○ ○ ○ ○ ○ |
| Uplifted | ○ ○ ○ ○ ○ |
| Creative | ○ ○ ○ ○ ○ |

**Ratings** ☆ ☆ ☆ ☆ ☆

# Strain

Grower _____  Date _____

Acquired _____  $ _____

| Indica | Hybrid | Sativa |

☐ Flower   ☐ Edible   ☐ Concentrate

**Symptoms Relieved**
_____
_____
_____
_____

Sweet · Fruity · Floral · Sour · Spicy · Earthy · Woodsy · Herbal

**Notes**
_____
_____
_____
_____
_____
_____

| Effects | Strength | | | | |
|---|---|---|---|---|---|
| Peaceful | ○ | ○ | ○ | ○ | ○ |
| Sleepy | ○ | ○ | ○ | ○ | ○ |
| Pain Relief | ○ | ○ | ○ | ○ | ○ |
| Hungry | ○ | ○ | ○ | ○ | ○ |
| Uplifted | ○ | ○ | ○ | ○ | ○ |
| Creative | ○ | ○ | ○ | ○ | ○ |

Ratings ☆ ☆ ☆ ☆ ☆

# Strain

Grower _____  Date _____

Acquired _____  $ _____

| Indica | Hybrid | Sativa |

☐ Flower  ☐ Edible  ☐ Concentrate

**Symptoms Relieved**
_____
_____
_____
_____
_____

Sweet / Floral / Spicy / Herbal / Woodsy / Earthy / Sour / Fruity

**Notes**
_____
_____
_____
_____
_____

| Effects | Strength |
|---|---|
| Peaceful | ○ ○ ○ ○ ○ |
| Sleepy | ○ ○ ○ ○ ○ |
| Pain Relief | ○ ○ ○ ○ ○ |
| Hungry | ○ ○ ○ ○ ○ |
| Uplifted | ○ ○ ○ ○ ○ |
| Creative | ○ ○ ○ ○ ○ |

**Ratings** ☆ ☆ ☆ ☆ ☆

# Strain

Grower _____  Date _____

Acquired _____  $ _____

|  Indica  |  Hybrid  |  Sativa  |

☐ Flower  ☐ Edible  ☐ Concentrate

**Symptoms Relieved**

_____
_____
_____
_____
_____

Flavor wheel: Sweet, Floral, Spicy, Herbal, Woodsy, Earthy, Sour, Fruity

**Notes**

_____
_____
_____
_____
_____
_____

| Effects | Strength | | | | |
|---|---|---|---|---|---|
| Peaceful | ○ | ○ | ○ | ○ | ○ |
| Sleepy | ○ | ○ | ○ | ○ | ○ |
| Pain Relief | ○ | ○ | ○ | ○ | ○ |
| Hungry | ○ | ○ | ○ | ○ | ○ |
| Uplifted | ○ | ○ | ○ | ○ | ○ |
| Creative | ○ | ○ | ○ | ○ | ○ |

**Ratings** ☆ ☆ ☆ ☆ ☆

# Strain

Grower _____  Date _____

Acquired _____  $ _____

| Indica | Hybrid | Sativa |

☐ Flower   ☐ Edible   ☐ Concentrate

**Symptoms Relieved**

_____
_____
_____
_____
_____

Sweet · Fruity · Floral · Sour · Spicy · Earthy · Herbal · Woodsy

**Notes**

_____
_____
_____
_____
_____
_____
_____

| Effects | Strength | | | | |
|---|---|---|---|---|---|
| Peaceful | ○ | ○ | ○ | ○ | ○ |
| Sleepy | ○ | ○ | ○ | ○ | ○ |
| Pain Relief | ○ | ○ | ○ | ○ | ○ |
| Hungry | ○ | ○ | ○ | ○ | ○ |
| Uplifted | ○ | ○ | ○ | ○ | ○ |
| Creative | ○ | ○ | ○ | ○ | ○ |

**Ratings** ☆ ☆ ☆ ☆ ☆

# Strain

Grower _____  Date _____

Acquired _____  $ _____

| Indica | Hybrid | Sativa |

☐ Flower   ☐ Edible   ☐ Concentrate

**Symptoms Relieved**

_____
_____
_____
_____

Sweet · Fruity · Floral · Sour · Spicy · Earthy · Herbal · Woodsy

**Notes**

_____
_____
_____
_____
_____
_____

| Effects | Strength | | | | |
|---|---|---|---|---|---|
| Peaceful | ○ | ○ | ○ | ○ | ○ |
| Sleepy | ○ | ○ | ○ | ○ | ○ |
| Pain Relief | ○ | ○ | ○ | ○ | ○ |
| Hungry | ○ | ○ | ○ | ○ | ○ |
| Uplifted | ○ | ○ | ○ | ○ | ○ |
| Creative | ○ | ○ | ○ | ○ | ○ |

**Ratings** ☆ ☆ ☆ ☆ ☆

# Strain

Grower _____  Date _____

Acquired _____  $ _____

| Indica | Hybrid | Sativa |

☐ Flower  ☐ Edible  ☐ Concentrate

**Symptoms Relieved**

_____
_____
_____
_____
_____

Sweet · Floral · Spicy · Herbal · Woodsy · Earthy · Sour · Fruity

**Notes**

_____
_____
_____
_____
_____
_____

| Effects | Strength | | | | |
|---|---|---|---|---|---|
| Peaceful | ○ | ○ | ○ | ○ | ○ |
| Sleepy | ○ | ○ | ○ | ○ | ○ |
| Pain Relief | ○ | ○ | ○ | ○ | ○ |
| Hungry | ○ | ○ | ○ | ○ | ○ |
| Uplifted | ○ | ○ | ○ | ○ | ○ |
| Creative | ○ | ○ | ○ | ○ | ○ |

**Ratings** ☆ ☆ ☆ ☆ ☆

# Strain

Grower _____   Date _____

Acquired _____   $ _____

| Indica | Hybrid | Sativa |

☐ Flower   ☐ Edible   ☐ Concentrate

**Symptoms Relieved**

_____
_____
_____
_____

Flavor wheel: Sweet, Floral, Spicy, Herbal, Woodsy, Earthy, Sour, Fruity

**Notes**

_____
_____
_____
_____
_____
_____

| Effects | Strength |
|---|---|
| Peaceful | ○ ○ ○ ○ ○ |
| Sleepy | ○ ○ ○ ○ ○ |
| Pain Relief | ○ ○ ○ ○ ○ |
| Hungry | ○ ○ ○ ○ ○ |
| Uplifted | ○ ○ ○ ○ ○ |
| Creative | ○ ○ ○ ○ ○ |

**Ratings** ☆ ☆ ☆ ☆ ☆

# Strain

Grower _____  Date _____

Acquired _____  $ _____

|   Indica   |   Hybrid   |   Sativa   |

☐ Flower   ☐ Edible   ☐ Concentrate

**Symptoms Relieved**

_____
_____
_____
_____
_____

Sweet · Floral · Spicy · Herbal · Woodsy · Earthy · Sour · Fruity

**Notes**

_____
_____
_____
_____
_____

| Effects | Strength | | | | |
|---|---|---|---|---|---|
| Peaceful | ○ | ○ | ○ | ○ | ○ |
| Sleepy | ○ | ○ | ○ | ○ | ○ |
| Pain Relief | ○ | ○ | ○ | ○ | ○ |
| Hungry | ○ | ○ | ○ | ○ | ○ |
| Uplifted | ○ | ○ | ○ | ○ | ○ |
| Creative | ○ | ○ | ○ | ○ | ○ |

**Ratings** ☆ ☆ ☆ ☆ ☆

# Strain

Grower _____    Date _____

Acquired _____    $ _____

|   Indica   |   Hybrid   |   Sativa   |

☐ Flower    ☐ Edible    ☐ Concentrate

**Symptoms Relieved**

_____
_____
_____
_____

Sweet / Fruity / Floral / Sour / Spicy / Earthy / Woodsy / Herbal

**Notes**

_____
_____
_____
_____
_____
_____

| Effects | Strength |
|---|---|
| Peaceful | ○ ○ ○ ○ ○ |
| Sleepy | ○ ○ ○ ○ ○ |
| Pain Relief | ○ ○ ○ ○ ○ |
| Hungry | ○ ○ ○ ○ ○ |
| Uplifted | ○ ○ ○ ○ ○ |
| Creative | ○ ○ ○ ○ ○ |

**Ratings** ☆ ☆ ☆ ☆ ☆

# Strain

Grower _____  Date _____

Acquired _____  $ _____

| Indica | Hybrid | Sativa |

☐ Flower   ☐ Edible   ☐ Concentrate

**Symptoms Relieved**

_____
_____
_____
_____
_____

Sweet · Floral · Spicy · Herbal · Woodsy · Earthy · Sour · Fruity

**Notes**

_____
_____
_____
_____
_____

| Effects | Strength | | | | |
|---|---|---|---|---|---|
| Peaceful | ○ | ○ | ○ | ○ | ○ |
| Sleepy | ○ | ○ | ○ | ○ | ○ |
| Pain Relief | ○ | ○ | ○ | ○ | ○ |
| Hungry | ○ | ○ | ○ | ○ | ○ |
| Uplifted | ○ | ○ | ○ | ○ | ○ |
| Creative | ○ | ○ | ○ | ○ | ○ |

**Ratings** ☆ ☆ ☆ ☆ ☆

# Strain

Grower _____  Date _____

Acquired _____  $ _____

| Indica | Hybrid | Sativa |

☐ Flower   ☐ Edible   ☐ Concentrate

**Symptoms Relieved**

_____
_____
_____
_____
_____

Sweet  Fruity  Floral  Sour  Spicy  Earthy  Herbal  Woodsy

**Notes**

_____
_____
_____
_____
_____
_____

| Effects | Strength | | | | |
|---|---|---|---|---|---|
| Peaceful | ○ | ○ | ○ | ○ | ○ |
| Sleepy | ○ | ○ | ○ | ○ | ○ |
| Pain Relief | ○ | ○ | ○ | ○ | ○ |
| Hungry | ○ | ○ | ○ | ○ | ○ |
| Uplifted | ○ | ○ | ○ | ○ | ○ |
| Creative | ○ | ○ | ○ | ○ | ○ |

**Ratings** ☆ ☆ ☆ ☆ ☆

# Strain

Grower _____  Date _____

Acquired _____  $ _____

| Indica | Hybrid | Sativa |

☐ Flower  ☐ Edible  ☐ Concentrate

**Symptoms Relieved**
_____
_____
_____
_____
_____

Sweet · Floral · Spicy · Herbal · Woodsy · Earthy · Sour · Fruity

**Notes**
_____
_____
_____
_____
_____
_____
_____

| Effects | Strength |
|---|---|
| Peaceful | ○ ○ ○ ○ ○ |
| Sleepy | ○ ○ ○ ○ ○ |
| Pain Relief | ○ ○ ○ ○ ○ |
| Hungry | ○ ○ ○ ○ ○ |
| Uplifted | ○ ○ ○ ○ ○ |
| Creative | ○ ○ ○ ○ ○ |

**Ratings** ☆ ☆ ☆ ☆ ☆

# Strain

Grower _____     Date _____

Acquired _____     $ _____

| Indica | Hybrid | Sativa |

☐ Flower    ☐ Edible    ☐ Concentrate

**Symptoms Relieved**

_____
_____
_____
_____

Sweet · Fruity · Floral · Sour · Spicy · Earthy · Woodsy · Herbal

**Notes**

_____
_____
_____
_____
_____
_____

| Effects | Strength |
|---|---|
| Peaceful | ○ ○ ○ ○ ○ |
| Sleepy | ○ ○ ○ ○ ○ |
| Pain Relief | ○ ○ ○ ○ ○ |
| Hungry | ○ ○ ○ ○ ○ |
| Uplifted | ○ ○ ○ ○ ○ |
| Creative | ○ ○ ○ ○ ○ |

Ratings ☆ ☆ ☆ ☆ ☆

# Strain

Grower _____  Date _____

Acquired _____  $ _____

|  Indica  |  Hybrid  |  Sativa  |

☐ Flower   ☐ Edible   ☐ Concentrate

**Symptoms Relieved**

_____
_____
_____
_____
_____

Sweet · Fruity · Floral · Sour · Spicy · Earthy · Herbal · Woodsy

**Notes**

_____
_____
_____
_____
_____

| Effects | Strength | | | | |
|---|---|---|---|---|---|
| Peaceful | ○ | ○ | ○ | ○ | ○ |
| Sleepy | ○ | ○ | ○ | ○ | ○ |
| Pain Relief | ○ | ○ | ○ | ○ | ○ |
| Hungry | ○ | ○ | ○ | ○ | ○ |
| Uplifted | ○ | ○ | ○ | ○ | ○ |
| Creative | ○ | ○ | ○ | ○ | ○ |

**Ratings** ☆ ☆ ☆ ☆ ☆

# Strain

Grower _____    Date _____

Acquired _____    $ _____

|   Indica    |    Hybrid    |    Sativa   |
|---|---|---|

☐ Flower   ☐ Edible   ☐ Concentrate

**Symptoms Relieved**

_____
_____
_____
_____

Sweet · Floral · Spicy · Herbal · Woodsy · Earthy · Sour · Fruity

**Notes**

_____
_____
_____
_____
_____
_____

| Effects | Strength | | | | |
|---|---|---|---|---|---|
| Peaceful | ○ | ○ | ○ | ○ | ○ |
| Sleepy | ○ | ○ | ○ | ○ | ○ |
| Pain Relief | ○ | ○ | ○ | ○ | ○ |
| Hungry | ○ | ○ | ○ | ○ | ○ |
| Uplifted | ○ | ○ | ○ | ○ | ○ |
| Creative | ○ | ○ | ○ | ○ | ○ |

**Ratings** ☆ ☆ ☆ ☆ ☆

# Strain

Grower _____  Date _____

Acquired _____  $ _____

|   Indica   |   Hybrid   |   Sativa   |
|------------|------------|------------|

☐ Flower  ☐ Edible  ☐ Concentrate

**Symptoms Relieved**

_____
_____
_____
_____
_____

Sweet · Floral · Spicy · Herbal · Woodsy · Earthy · Sour · Fruity

**Notes**

_____
_____
_____
_____
_____
_____

| Effects | Strength | | | | |
|---|---|---|---|---|---|
| Peaceful | ○ | ○ | ○ | ○ | ○ |
| Sleepy | ○ | ○ | ○ | ○ | ○ |
| Pain Relief | ○ | ○ | ○ | ○ | ○ |
| Hungry | ○ | ○ | ○ | ○ | ○ |
| Uplifted | ○ | ○ | ○ | ○ | ○ |
| Creative | ○ | ○ | ○ | ○ | ○ |

**Ratings** ☆ ☆ ☆ ☆ ☆

# Strain

Grower _____  Date _____

Acquired _____  $ _____

| Indica | Hybrid | Sativa |

☐ Flower  ☐ Edible  ☐ Concentrate

**Symptoms Relieved**

_____
_____
_____
_____
_____

Sweet
Fruity    Floral
Sour    Spicy
Earthy    Herbal
Woodsy

**Notes**

_____
_____
_____
_____
_____

| Effects | Strength |
|---|---|
| Peaceful | ○ ○ ○ ○ ○ |
| Sleepy | ○ ○ ○ ○ ○ |
| Pain Relief | ○ ○ ○ ○ ○ |
| Hungry | ○ ○ ○ ○ ○ |
| Uplifted | ○ ○ ○ ○ ○ |
| Creative | ○ ○ ○ ○ ○ |

**Ratings** ☆ ☆ ☆ ☆ ☆

# Strain

Grower _____  Date _____

Acquired _____  $ _____

| Indica | Hybrid | Sativa |

☐ Flower   ☐ Edible   ☐ Concentrate

Sweet
Fruity   Floral
Sour   Spicy
Earthy   Herbal
Woodsy

**Symptoms Relieved**

_____
_____
_____
_____
_____

**Notes**

_____
_____
_____
_____
_____
_____

| Effects | Strength |
|---|---|
| Peaceful | ○ ○ ○ ○ ○ |
| Sleepy | ○ ○ ○ ○ ○ |
| Pain Relief | ○ ○ ○ ○ ○ |
| Hungry | ○ ○ ○ ○ ○ |
| Uplifted | ○ ○ ○ ○ ○ |
| Creative | ○ ○ ○ ○ ○ |

**Ratings** ☆ ☆ ☆ ☆ ☆

# Strain

Grower _____   Date _____

Acquired _____   $ _____

| Indica | Hybrid | Sativa |

☐ Flower   ☐ Edible   ☐ Concentrate

Sweet · Floral · Spicy · Herbal · Woodsy · Earthy · Sour · Fruity

**Symptoms Relieved**

_____
_____
_____
_____

**Notes**

_____
_____
_____
_____
_____

| Effects | Strength | | | | |
|---|---|---|---|---|---|
| Peaceful | ○ | ○ | ○ | ○ | ○ |
| Sleepy | ○ | ○ | ○ | ○ | ○ |
| Pain Relief | ○ | ○ | ○ | ○ | ○ |
| Hungry | ○ | ○ | ○ | ○ | ○ |
| Uplifted | ○ | ○ | ○ | ○ | ○ |
| Creative | ○ | ○ | ○ | ○ | ○ |

**Ratings** ☆ ☆ ☆ ☆ ☆

www.ingramcontent.com/pod-product-compliance
Lightning Source LLC
Chambersburg PA
CBHW021831170526
45157CB00007B/2757